Writing Away the Demons

Stories of Creative Coping
Through Transformative Writing

Writing Away the Demons

Stories of Creative Coping Through Transformative Writing

Sherry Reiter, PhD, LCSW, PTR/M-S
and
Contributors

Foreword by David Read Johnson, PhD, RDT-BCT

NORTH STAR PRESS OF ST. CLOUD, INC.
St. Cloud, Minnesota

ISBN: 978-0-87839-329-9

First Edition, April 15, 2009

Updated 2015

Printed in the United States of America

Published by
North Star Press of St. Cloud, Inc
St. Cloud, Minnesota

www.northstarpress.com

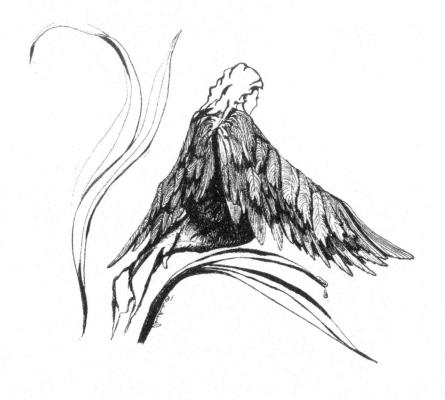

This book is dedicated to my clients, students, and colleagues who have courageously and generously shared their stories and made this book possible. "I saw the angel in the marble and carved till I set him free," wrote Michaelangelo. So has each author wielded the pen to liberate the creative spirit within. Each writer has discovered that words have the power to call upon angels and banish demons. Through writing, the self recognizes its identity with greater definition, harvests its wisdom, and wrestles with challenges, transforming them into building blocks of growth.

S.R.

~ • ~

Acknowledgements

I want to acknowledge, in addition to the authors, the host of angels who have been vital in the creation of *Writing Away the Demons*. My gratitude goes to Maryellen Bova for inspiring its conception. My deep thanks to Emily Blumenfeld and Ross Laird; your editorial expertise and kind support meant more to me than I can express. I felt fortunate to work with Malka Barshishat, the talented artist whose work graces this book. A special thank-you also to Dr. David Read Johnson for his foreword, as well as for providing me with a space at The Institutes for the Arts in Psychotherapy in New York City, where my work has flourished in the past decade. I truly appreciated the support and comments from readers Ann Forcier and Gladys Foxe. And to my dear friends and family, your encouragement and faith sustained me during the three-year period during which this book was written. Lastly, my thanks to North Star Press, for recognizing the value of this work, and using their expertise to produce the book you now hold in your hand.

TABLE OF CONTENTS

Foreword
David Read Johnson, PhD, RDT-BCT
viii

Introduction
The Ten Principles of Transformative Writing
Sherry Reiter, PhD, LCSW, PTR/M-S
1

Chapter 1
The Woman Who Plowed Verses
Linda Lanza
18

Chapter 2
The Poem That Was Snake Medicine
Preston H. Hood, III
42

Chapter 3
Greetings from Cancerland
Alysa Cummings
62

Chapter 4
The Journal That Was an Anchor
Joel Gabriel
77

Chapter 5
Tír na mBan
Maryellen Bova
97

Chapter 6
The Poem That Was a Prayer
Sister Mary Sullivan
111

Chapter 7
The Woman Who Went Nightfishing
Nadia Antonopoulos
130

Chapter 8
The Words That Built a Fortress
Richard Fireman
150

Chapter 9
The Woman Who Changed a Triangle into a Circle
Barbara Bethea
168

Chapter 10
The Woman Who Built a Labyrinth with Words
Susan Riback
182

Chapter 11
The Words That Were Magic Pebbles
Nancy Bengis Friedman
200

Chapter 12
Notes from the Back of the Class
Mark Auster
218

Chapter 13
The Journal That Was a Reservoir of Tears
Leah Tamar
237

Conclusion
256

End Notes
260

Recommended Reading for the Writer in You
275

~ • ~

Foreword

There is a bridge between the present and my past. I call her memory, and over her I travel back and forth, my home now there, then here, seeking comfort against the uncertainties that press on me. With her, I revisit the kind gestures, the warm embraces, the belly laughs that graced my life along the way and that help me face the rising edge of time which greets me each morning.

But I also travel back along that bridge into darker corners, and I don't know why. Surely I should heed the signs of warning and calls to turn back that have been placed along the way, by me, after previous upsetting forays! Why do I return to these moments or months of grief or fear or violence, that raised fist, the shameful disrobing, those awful words, which sliced my heart in two? Let memory fade. Let the day begin anew. Let me be buoyed by the possibilities of the future, not the hard facts of the past. Besides, *I have no words for what happened to me*, and even if I were to find them, *I cannot imagine that anyone will be interested* in another sad story. And even if they were interested, *no one can really understand what I went through* because they were not there. I was alone. I remain alone. I remain alone except that sometimes I can see, like flocks of birds in the sky, gatherings of words swirling about me and I reach out and pull one, then another to me,

xi

clothing myself in a fabric of words, keeping close company. In this way, I can make sense of what happened—what I felt and thought and risked and lost and learned. This helps time resume again—for it has stopped of late—and I can leave this bridge for a while.

As a clinical psychologist who has worked with trauma survivors for more than three decades, I have watched many individuals who have paused on the bridge. So I was very interested in reading the words of the thirteen souls in this book who describe their passages between past and present: yes, I see the outpouring of narrative, the care over details, the sudden stop to let confusion pass, and of course the weight of grief and fear carried by each sentence. These stories of living through alcoholism, Vietnam, cancer, violence, imprisonment, and multiple sclerosis bring me again and again to the same question: *Why me? How can I survive this?*

Preston or Maryellen or Nancy and the others provide their answers, and I feel myself wishing to banish memory so that none of this struggle is needed, but I read on nevertheless, because these are good stories, amazing stories, written to be read. Read by the authors themselves, suddenly switching places with themselves, utterly surprised by the very words that came from their hand moments before. Read by Dr. Sherry Reiter, who gave them encouragement and the validation that their experience was important. And now read by me, book in my lap, memory again knocking on my door! This process cannot end with me, I must share their messages with someone else!

And that is you! I am certain that this book will command your attention. Like the people who broke out of prison by digging a tunnel with spoons, these authors have broken out of their prisons of memory with pens. This is not a book about transformative writing; this book *is* transformative writing! The authors write deeply and beautifully about their experiences and their healing process, illustrating directly both their resiliency and the power of creative writing. Dr. Reiter provides an excellent overview of the therapeutic effects of writing in the first chapter, noting ten principles derived from a broad range of sources such as anthropology, psychology, mythology, cognitive science, and the arts. Her graceful introductions to each chapter are followed by insightful reflections afterwards that highlight important elements in each author's narrative. Throughout, one feels the power of transformational writing in altering people's relationship to their own history. All thirteen stories are gripping, and once begun, they are hard to put down. They are at times short story, autobiography, and pages from a secret diary; each one entirely unique. One is left with respect for the misfortunes possible within the human condition, and awe for the individuals who can overcome them.

There is a bridge between the present and my past. I call her memory, and after reading this book, I think I can call her friend.

David Read Johnson, PhD, RDT-BCT
Director, Institutes for the Arts in Psychotherapy, New York, New York
Co-Director, Post-Traumatic Stress Center, New Haven, Connecticut
Assoc. Clinical Prof., Dept. of Psychiatry, Yale University School of Medicine

~ Introduction ~

The Ten Principles of Transformative Writing

W riting Away the Demons: Stories of Creative Coping through Transformative Writing shares the experiences of thirteen men and women who have benefited from the power of personal writing. Although this is not a how-to book, it is a primer of transformative writing, a collection of stories to illustrate the benefits of writing for psychological health and well-being.

Confronted with crisis, scientists tell us there are three responses to stress: fight, flight, or freeze.[1] This book features a different response to stress —the creative coping response of writing. Transformative writing is a way of completing those incomplete traumatic responses. It is, in fact, a way of creatively clearing one's way through the brushfire, and discovering a path forward, past the place we felt unable to go. By finishing the poem and by telling the story we complete our frozen and disoriented responses. A place that was previously dark is illuminated.

The term "demon" as it is used in this book is not an evil spirit that takes possession of your body. It connotes a powerful upheaval that seems to take over one's existence. It generally refers to an external force, or an uninvited situation into which the person is thrust. For example, Linda lives with the fury of an alcoholic partner. Or it may be an internal force, either

1

physical or psychological. For example, Alysa must cope with the diagnosis of breast cancer. Whether the stressors are external or internal, strong emotions are triggered. Crises in our lives are often surrounded by dark forces of confusion, fear, and anger. However, the greatest weapon to fight the dark may be the creative imagination. No fight, no flight—just write!

Perhaps you are thinking that it is far too simplistic to suggest that our problems can be "written away" simply by putting pen to paper. And you are absolutely correct. In fact, instead of escaping or distancing oneself from the demon, writing provides a safe meeting place of encounter. In that encounter, the relationship between oneself and one's problem starts to change. Is there struggle in the process? Sometimes. However, people who write for their own well-being frequently report experiencing the joy and relief of honest unbridled self-expression and catharsis. Writing offers an effective, safe, and creative coping mechanism.

No one is immune from dealing with illness, loss, and trauma. Nietzsche, the German philosopher, once said, "That which does not kill me makes me stronger."[2] The demons in our lives are wrestling partners. Such a partner has the potential of ultimately strengthening us. Historically, it is interesting to note that not all demons were considered evil. In ancient Greece, the demon was called a "daemon," and it was believed that each person had his/her own spirit guide or guardian to assist in the life journey.[3] The daemon was a benevolent instructor. Only if pure of heart, the individual could open himself/herself to the daemon's wisdom.

All art is borne out of struggle. Edward Hirsch writes about angels and demons as sources of the creative imagination: "They come only when something is at risk, when the soul is imperiled and pushes against its limits, when death is possible. The struggle will pierce one's soul to the depths, and at the same time provide access to the higher self."[4] The mystery, passion, and raw emotion fueling the creative act has been termed "duende" by the Spanish poet, Federico Garcia Lorca.[5] When duende possesses its creative host, a dancer or singer or writer may appear to be in a trance. Angel, demon, and duende all have the magical power to make something visible that was previously invisible through the process of writing.

Transformative Writing

We tend to lose our balance in life because we sometimes respond to our life experience with extremes of emotion—fear, sorrow, anger, and even joy. Creative "Righting" (a term coined at The Creative Righting Center in New York City) is based on the simple belief that reading and writing are beneficial to one's psychological health and emotional balance. Freud's "talking cure" and the "writing cure" are built on the same premise: self-expression and disinhibition are healing factors. In Freud's time, only the wealthy and upper middle class were well educated and had the ability to write. With the coming of mandatory education, writing is a tool that belongs to everyone.

You may be asking, what is "transformative writing"? Simply put, transformative writing is the intentional use of writing for psychological change and well-being. As Shaun McNiff, a leading scholar on the expressive arts, says, "Words become agents of transformation, shamanic horses that carry expression and transport people to change."[6]

Although some people think of transformative writing as a new age modality, transformative language is as ancient as prayer. Transformative writing takes many forms and also goes by these names: "writing therapy," "poetry therapy," "bibliotherapy," "journaling" and "journal therapy."[7] The writer can dialogue with the self. One part of the self asks a question, and another part of the self answers. Possibilities for personal growth and healing multiply when the power of transformative language is engaged.

Modern researchers support the premise of a self-righting mechanism that is similar to the body's innate ability to heal wounds. Just as a plant will naturally turn toward light, given the opportunity and resources to "right" (balance) oneself, human beings possess an amazing capacity for self-healing.

Dr. James Pennebaker (1990)[8] conducted the first landmark study to link "disinhibition" or "opening up" on paper to greater physical and emotional health. Pennebaker asked students to write their deepest thoughts and feelings about the most traumatic event in their lives for a short period on four consecutive days. Subjects in this group showed significant decline in doctor visits for two to four months after the study, in comparison with control subjects, who were asked to write about trivial subjects. A significant increase in the experimental subjects' immune function, and ability to withstand infection was noted.

Researchers Stephen Lepore and Joshua Smyth edited the most recent comprehensive collection of studies in the field (*The Writing Cure*, 2002).[9] Writing affects heart rate, blood pressure, and your immune system, and the power of writing from the heart results in stress reduction and the restoration of emotional equilibrium. When we write from the heart, we impact mind, body, and spirit. Spirit and mind are difficult to quantify, but the body registers our stress level and records disturbances on a biological plane. Laboratory tests are able to document the effects of writing on a cellular level. Although more conclusive studies need to be done, there is substantial evidence that writing about one's feelings and telling one's story is a step toward psychological and physical well being.

Each person who has contributed to *Writing Away the Demons* has found their way to a paper and pen on their own. It is an innate ability of humans to find a way to express what cannot be expressed in any other way. From our earliest beginnings, humankind has creatively expressed emotion through music, art, and dance. Archaeologists who have found ancient hieroglyphics on cave walls believe that writing was the last art form to develop, some 10,000 years ago.

Today writing is the most easily accessible of all the art forms. Journal therapist Kathleen Adams calls writing "the seventy-nine-cent therapist,"[10] available at any time of day or night, as close as your nearest paper and pen or pencil. This is not to suggest that self-guided writing takes the place of a therapist; a therapist may be extremely helpful and is sometimes necessary in the process of healing and personal growth. But no therapist can be available twenty-four hours a day. Although writing may take place in the counseling space, particularly if the person is working with a poetry therapist (yes, there is such a thing as a poetry therapist!), most of the writing samples in this book were done in the privacy of each person's home at a time of their own choosing.

Your writing is your own truth as you are experiencing it at that moment. Even if you do not understand what you are feeling at the time, when you read and re-read your own writing, you are most likely to "crack the code," and discover new meaning. Those little black squiggles on the paper have an extraordinary ability to bring us to a new level of self-knowledge and awareness.

There are ten basic concepts that can assist us in understanding why writing may facilitate transformation. The same principles that were used in ancient healing apply to the current practice of creative "righting" or writing for emotional balance. These important healing principles have withstood the tests of time.

1. MASTERY

Writing is a form of empowerment. From toddlerhood on, words are the structure through which you communicate your wants and needs. Not surprisingly, words are also the building blocks for prayer and magic spells. The ability to use or apply language is a fundamental tool, instinctive to humans. Feelings of pain, fear, anger, and confusion start to transform when we have the courage to identify the demons, externalize them onto the page, and view them from a different perspective. When thoughts and feelings remain formless and invisible, the demon may dance in the shadow of your mind. But when pen is put to paper, and you hold that paper up to the light, your honesty and courage overpowers the dark.

In many civilizations, there was a strong belief that to name someone or something was to magically possess it or have power over it. In ancient Egypt, for example, the name not only expressed the identity, it was thought to be the essence of a person's being, and was believed to be essential for survival.[11] Therefore, newborns' names often contained the name of a powerful god. Ancient Egyptians also had a custom of writing their enemies' names on a stone cuneiform tablet and then smashing it as a symbolic gesture of victory over their enemies.[12] This magical thinking substituted the word for the actual object and incorporated wish fulfillment.

Remember the story of Helen Keller?[13] When her teacher first spells out W-A-T-E-R, a whole new world opens up. Helen is deliriously happy and runs from object to object as her teacher spells out its name. With her new mastery, she is able to organize her world and understand that each thing has its place. Similarly, writing can help you to identify and organize thoughts and feelings. How does making little black squiggles on a sheet of paper help with the wrestling of demons? If you can reduce the demon to the size of a page, certainly you are much bigger than the problem itself!

2. RITUAL

Whenever human beings have been faced with change, whether alone or in groups, we create rituals to give significance to life passages.[14] Rituals acknowledge deep feelings, as well as the need for connection to self, community, and the sacred. Writing circles lend themselves beautifully to this ritual, and are a natural re-creation of ancient healing circles where words were used for prayer and dialogue with the sacred.

Traditionally, humans have always created rites of passage for birth, puberty, menopause, marriage, and death. During these transitional phases, the individual is leaving one world, and about to enter a new one, but is not yet there. Rituals offer us meaningful activities that reduce feelings of anxiety, depression, and helplessness.

The word "journal" comes from the French journée: day.[15] In the seventeenth century it meant a day's travel or journey as well as a record of the day's events. It was a form of predictability as well as change. Taking time out to write about your life in a journal may be considered a rite or ritual in which you take the time to acknowledge the smaller, ongoing transitions that life demands. Choosing a special place that can be visited regularly enhances the writing ritual.

Ancient rituals often used drumming or other percussion instruments to induce an altered state of consciousness. In a relaxed or altered state, the inner world of symbols may be easily accessed. Rituals may also be used prior to the writing journey; some individuals choose to light a candle, meditate, dance, or play music. Such rituals provide portals that enable you to enter into a new state of consciousness.

3. SAFETY

James Dickey once called poetry the "last refuge of non-manipulative language."[16] When language is not focused on communicating with others, it may function as a way of communicating with the self. Because this communication is done in private, without any need to please or impress others, it is free of judgment and absolutely safe. The words are for the writer's eyes alone. Only the writer decides if they are to be shared with a friend, a partner, or a therapist.

This is not about becoming a Danielle Steele or James Michener. When writing for oneself, it is about the process of creative "righting," not the product of creative writing. It is essential that the writer grant himself/herself permission to be authentic and imperfect. Nothing that one writes can be wrong. The harsh inner critic that many of us have must be banned from one's journal, otherwise the safety is compromised, writing becomes guarded, and authenticity is no longer possible.

The process of writing is about creating an intimate relationship—with one's self. Like any intimate relationship, confidentiality, honesty, and the permission to be in a judgment-free space are required. Most of us don't live in such a place. We have to create it. The white space of a lined journal awaits you.

4. WITNESSING

The word "witness" is from "wit," signifying knowledge or intelligence. Prior to it becoming a legal term in the 1800s, it meant an attestation of fact or event based on personal knowledge. Recording your thoughts and feelings provides a testament to your life experience. Like all humans, you almost never see yourself completely and objectively, unless you are able to videotape yourself, sit back, and observe yourself from a different perspective. When you write, through the process of externalization, your invisible thoughts and feelings become visible. Once on paper, your observing ego can view the situation. The observing ego may be thought of as a part of the self that sees objectively.

7

Writing makes witnessing possible, and gives you another vantage point from which you can view the situation. When you write your feelings in a journal, you are expressing and containing those feelings at the same time. When you read the words, you are witnessing your own evidence—evidence that you have procured through your own self-knowledge and lived experience.

With witnessing, come new observations, reflections and sometimes a new perspective. You can return to your thoughts and feelings whenever you choose. Your writing is a semi-permanent recording, yours to save, erase, edit and re-read as often as you choose.

If you are like most people in this technological age, you live life at warp speed. The rapid pace may distort the way you view your own story, somewhat like a photo that is blurred because the photographer is in motion. To further complicate selp-perception, you are vulnerable to how others view you. You began as an adjunct to your parents' story. Family, friends, and others you meet will, no doubt, want to share their perspective of your life story. Sometimes this is valuable; sometimes it is destructive. No doubt, sometimes it is confusing.

When the mirror of self-reflection is muddy, clarify by putting pen to paper. Trust the gift of self-knowledge. Trust your own "wit," the keen sense of "knowing" that is innate to your most authentic self.

You can return to your thoughts and feelings whenever you choose. Your writing is a semi-permanent recording, yours to save or erase, as you choose.

5. FREEDOM/POETIC LICENSE

One of the great psychotherapists, Virginia Satir, wrote about the "five freedoms"[17]
- the freedom to see and hear what is present instead of what should be, was, or will be;
- the freedom to feel what you feel instead of what you "should" feel;
- the freedom to say what you think and feel instead of what you ought to think and feel;

- the freedom to ask for what you want instead of always waiting for permission;
- the freedom to take risks on your own behalf instead of choosing to be only "secure" and not rocking the boat.

You are entitled to these five freedoms. Do you know who issues your poetic license? You are the only one who can author-ize your own "rightings"!

Writing is self-directed. That means that the writer controls the intensity or depth, the pace, the duration (amount of time), and the subject matter. The person decides on the form. Shall it be a journal entry, a poem, a short story? Writing offers a range of possibility. Language may be concrete or figurative and metaphoric. The public face shown to the world may be very different from the private one. Freedom gives the writer the space to claim shadow aspects of self. Anais Nin wrote about the false persona she created for friends and reflected that the gay, receptive, sympathetic personality "had to have its other existence somewhere. In the diary, I could re-establish the balance. Here I could be depressed, angry, despairing, discouraged. I could let out all my demons."[18] The writer may approach the literature from an intellectual viewpoint or an emotional viewpoint, or both. Words may be used to reveal or conceal.

It is the nature of the poetic to be paradoxical, and large enough to hold contradiction. "Do I contradict myself? Yes, I contradict myself. I am large. I contain multitudes," said Walt Whitman.[19] Writing is a wonderful opportunity to exercise your five freedoms. There is no expense involved. In fact, if you do not issue your own poetic license—if you shove down your thoughts and feelings and eat your own words, you are likely to pay a much steeper price in terms of your health, which leads us to the next principle.

6. VENTING AND CONTAINMENT

According to Aristotle's theory of catharsis, the Greek dramas enabled audiences to vicariously experience such emotions as pity, guilt, and sorrow. Spectators of tragedies and comedies performed at Epidaurus would cleanse themselves through their laughter and tears as they participated in the Greek festival, said to last for several days at a time. Writing is the do-it-yourself version, requiring what may be only a few minutes of writing for cathartic relief.

Freud's "talking cure" is based on the idea that as the client spoke in the therapy session, repressed material from the subconscious would rise to the surface and the individual would be liberated from emotional conflict. Implicit within the talking cure is the importance of releasing words that serves to release feeling. Until the words are expressed, the feelings are repressed, which may result in tension, frustration, or depression. Or in a psychosomatic illness, as suggested by psychiatrist Jack J. Leedy who often stated, "An ulcer is a poem struggling to be born." [20]

There is a fifteenth century tale from Persia about a poet who went to a doctor complaining of depression and an inside full of knots.[21] The doctor asked whether he had composed a new poem lately that he had not recited or published. The poet said that he had such a poem inside him. The doctor had him recite it one—two— three times. He then told the poet "Be gone, you are cured. It was this poem that was tied up inside you. Now it has come forth in the open and you have found recovery."

Productive venting is done purposefully in writing therapy or journal therapy. The words are not simply released. They are simultaneously contained when a journal is used. Words symbolically leave the person and are transported to a place there they are safely held and may be revisited at any time in the future. Containment is as vital as expression. How the words are released, to whom they are released, and how the words are contained all contribute to safety, a sense of mastery, and poetic license.

The French writer Jean Cocteau kept a journal, *Opium: Diary of a Cure*, to help him through the pain and anguish of recovery. The experience "would have dissolved leaving no other trace behind except a deep depression, if a fountain pen had not given it a direction, relief and shape . . . Thought made flesh."[22]

7. THE MAGIC OF THE POETIC
Transformation of Time, Space, and Matter

As far back as the fourth millennium B.C.E., Egyptian chants were written on papyrus by the healer.[23] The words were dissolved into a solution that could then be physically ingested, so that the power of the words could take effect immediately. In the modern version of creative "righting," when you write, you slow down to take in your own words and similarly "digest" them, integrating thought, feeling, and experience. Thoughts and feelings that were previously invisible become visible through externalization. Time, space, and matter shift or change in the act of putting pen to paper.

By its very nature, writing is a time shifter, expanding or contracting the moment as needed. In the process of writing you are re-discovering that which you already know. When time-shifting, you return to an original experience by writing it and then reading it, "milking" the moment for all the richness we can extract from it. Writing enables you to return to those moments, both ugly and beautiful. The traumatized person may need to return to moments of pain and catastrophe, which are often sudden and swift and have not been processed completely by the brain. In returning to the moment of trauma, the writer expands the moment in order to process and integrate what could not be integrated before. Memory helps us to know who we are and where we have been.

When we write about hopes and dreams, we are time-shifting into the future. Some theories suggest that purposeful thought process paired with the motor activity required in writing is a precursor of action in the real world.[24] The poetic imagination permits us to visit the past, present, and future. In writing, we are capable of manipulating time, space, and matter. A personal playspace is literally created with building blocks of words.

The Poetic Mind

Regardless of the form the writing may take—storytelling, journal writing, or poetry, it is the poetic aspects within all of these forms that distinguish their use in transformational growth and healing. Psychologist Daniel

Goleman has helped us to understand that "the logic of the emotional mind is associative. It takes elements that symbolize a reality or trigger a memory of it, to be the same as that reality. That is why similes, metaphors, and images speak directly to the emotional mind . . ."[25] There is much to be learned in life that is not rational or logical. Creative writing is a modality that can help you to access your creative emotional intelligence and imagination.

Storytelling is one of the oldest, most comforting forms, having its roots in oral tradition. Writer Isak Dineson once said, "All sorrows can be borne if you put them into a story or tell a story about them."[26] Each contributor in Writing Away the Demons tells his or her story and shares excerpts of the writing used to transform their experience.

Several of the authors have chosen to write in poetry, a primary language that uses our visual inner eye, much as we do in dreams. If dreams are the royal road to the unconscious, as Freud suggested, then metaphor is the drawbridge allowing us to enter a deeper realm of feeling and thought.

Both dreams and poetry use the same psychological principles of imagery, condensation, and displacement.[27] All three mechanisms rely on poetic magic. Through imagery, we suddenly see what was not there before. Through condensation, much is distilled into little. Through displacement, the energy of a feeling or thought goes to a place we don't expect, similar to our surprise when the rabbit comes out of the magician's hat.

Both avenues explore dreams and the imaginal world. Although Freud is generally thought to have discovered dream interpretation, ancient healing rituals used this technique thousands of years ago. Imagery—visual, auditory, tactile, olfactory, and taste—were all used in shamanic ceremonies.

Simile and metaphor are found not only in ancient healing chants but in the prayers currently used in religious institutions. Perhaps the most beloved hymn of all time is Psalm 23: "The Lord is my shepherd; I shall not want . . ." Metaphor is derived from two ancient Greek words: "meta—meaning beyond, across, over, and "phor," meaning to carry, bring, or bear.[28] The word metaphor literally means " to carry across." It unites the realms of feeling and thought, inner life and outer life, the concrete and the invisible, the mundane and the sacred.

Poetry has often been called the language of the soul. For reasons we do not completely understand, poetry sometimes taps into a spiritual dimension or calls upon a Higher Power. Expression of the self may lead to the transpersonal beyond the self to cosmic, global, and spiritual concerns.

A powerful energy can be tapped into when people write. This energy is perceived like a force of nature; it is vast, powerful, and mysterious. Psychiatrist Silvano Arieti called it the "endocept."[29] He describes it as a form of unconscious or preconscious cognition of past experiences, memory traces and images of things and movements that acts as a springboard or cat- alyst for creative expression. Writer Gary Snyder may be referring to this same force, when he writes about an encounter with a "big mind" harvesting spirituality and creativity.[30] Regardless of what this force is called, it is clear that the "magic" of the poetic involves access to an energy that is transformative in its power.

8. CREATIVITY

"What we call the beginning is often the end
And to make an end is to make a beginning."
T.S. Eliot, "Little Gidding"

It is important to recognize that a creative being lives within each of us, whether we like it, recognize it, or live in denial of it. As writer/artist M.C. Richards states, "we must get out of its way, for it will give us no peace until we do."[31] An act of self is called for, whether in the form of art, writing, music, carpentry, cooking, or some other creative endeavor. This act of creating is a priceless gift that may be cherished privately or shared. For M.C. Richards, writer and potterer, it was, "An act of self, from me to you. From center to center . . . We must mean what we say from our innermost heart to the outermost galaxy . . ."[32]

Human beings are called on to reinvent themselves over and over again. Sometimes you do it without much thought. You adjust yourself in old and new relationships. You stretch—or shrink—to meet your own expectations, as well as the expectations of others. Friendships die, marriages fall

13

apart, careers end. You meet new friends, find new partners, create new homes, and start new jobs.

What gives us the power to renew ourselves? Our resilience shows itself in our creativity. Interestingly enough, within the human body itself, there are "poietic" organs, such as the spleen or the lymph system, where there is continuous creation of new blood cells. Currently, stem cells are of particular interest for their ability to create and regenerate.[33] This poiesis is creativity on a biological level.

On a psychological and spiritual level, creativity enables us to transcend our limitations. It kindles the imagination, fuels our dreams, and plants seeds of hope that are vital for our renewal. Writing expands our awareness by introducing new information, new images, and the juxtaposition of different ideas. When we write, our natural creativity finds new ways to view ourselves and the world. We renew ourselves, and in some sense, we are born again.

9. INTEGRATING PARTS INTO A WHOLE

According to scholar Wallace Bacon, literature is the author's act of interpreting the fragmented parts of the whole.[34] Accordingly, poetry may be viewed as the art of mending the cut tongue and severed hands, as writer Melissa Reed suggests, "an act of reconnecting speech, movement, image and action when the narrative act of coalescence cannot be performed, and when the story is too painful to tell."[35] In the act of telling the story, the writer reattaches the fragments to the whole and gains greater insight into life and nature. In mathematical terms, the whole is more than the sum of its parts. The eye and the I play essential roles in healing, wholing and the re-invention of self.

Implicit within the meaning of the word therapy is the Greek "theraput," a midwife who originally made way for Psyche's head.[36] As Christina Baldwin writes, "therapy means to stretch one's limbs, or consciousness, opening oneself to the imagery and activity of labor."[37] Baldwin invites both men and women to work from the dark underground of our deepest selves toward the light of greater consciousness. When we write, we attend to our own labors; we are birthing and healing ourselves. Different parts of the self

14

become active. In the relationship within your mind, you attend to the labors of nurturing the self through your own creative imagination. Writing is the process through which the relationship becomes tangible.

This idea is based on the assumption that you are capable of having a relationship with your own mind. From the "lighthouse"—a point of observation that is built into our consciousness, we are able to safely observe our lives. While one part observes, another part of the self writes. One part of the self asks questions. From the observing eye, you view the question and you attain perspective; another part of the self comes forth with answers. Through this dialogue with the self and its many parts, you grow and heal. Not surprisingly, the word heal comes from the root "hale" that means "to make whole."[38]

From the lighthouse window, you can observe the panoply of emotions and behaviors of your life; the pen becomes the funnel for all that you feel and permit yourself to express. The writing is your container, a ship bouncing on the waves of your emotions. And from these waters, re-birth takes place—sporadically, sometimes awkwardly and sometimes in pain, with the ultimate triumph of creation and transformation.

10. THEORY OF SELF AND RELATIONSHIPS
(Self-in-the-World)

The term "theory of self" is used to suggest a cohesive self-image in which the many aspects, voices and images connect to each other and form an integrated whole, as discussed in Principle 9. Once the self is cohesive, connection to the larger world is possible.

Relationship or connection is the ability to relate and connect with the larger world. It is an important concept of wellness that tribal groups have always embraced, usually through symbol, ritual, and ceremony.

The articulation of self or self-expression counters numbness and alienation, as does relating to significant others and the community at large. Those who struggle with their relations to other humans may choose to connect to a pet, the beauty of nature, or the Divine to counter feelings of disconnection.

15

A trauma victim's experience may constrict the inner world to two sole entities: the victim and the trauma. However, this tightly knit relationship can be permeated by expressions of caring, empathy, and the support of family and friends. Relationships and connection are essential for every human being to achieve psychological health and well being, especially in times of illness, trauma, and difficulties.

Gemstones

I have had the good fortune of meeting the contributors through my work at The Creative "Righting" Center in New York. The authors are my clients, former trainees, and colleagues. In my work as a therapist and poetry therapy trainer, I became mesmerized by the stories and writings that emerged in the process. I cherish these poem and story gems; they are like semi-precious stones slipped into my chest pocket. I take them out, reflect on them often, and am startled by their beauty, their vivid colors and authenticity. They are the unique offspring of each personality, and, although they always remain the property of the owner, shared reflection only seems to make them glow brighter.

Writing fulfills multiple psychological functions. First of all, many write for self-regulation of emotion and catharsis. Others write for clarification and organization. We may write and reread our writing for reflection and problem-solving. Writing strengthens the self-concept (self-image) through self-discovery, self-expression, self-nurturance, and affirmation of identity. Stimulation or play may be an objective. In a more serious vein, a person may write to bear witness, and for integration, particularly when trauma has occurred. Still others write to discover new information or connect with new aspects of the self, as well as the universe at large, including the Divine.

In the chapters that follow, you will meet the individuals who adapt the writing tool to creatively cope with their own unique life situations. Linda, in Chapter 1, writes to express her individuality, and her writings help to extricate her from an alcoholic husband. Preston, a veteran, writes to lay to rest the war memories that haunt him in Chapter 2. Alysa is a breast-cancer survivor who writes for a sense of mastery in Chapter 3. Joel, in Chapter 4, writes to create stability following the turbulent seas of childhood. Maryellen, in Chapter 5, writes to express her truth in a safe way, in spite of the fact that she lives in a house filled with danger. Sister Mary, in Chapter 6, is a nun who writes to access the Divine during a health crisis, while Nadia, in Chapter 7, writes to access the meaning of symbols in her subconscious to solve a riddle from her past.

Writing for self-affirmation and the articulation of identity plays a powerful role in many of the chapters. Rich, in Chapter 8, writes to protect himself and affirm his own boundaries while he watches his mother die of Alzheimer's. In Chapter 9, Barbara, a surivor of domestic violence, writes to reclaim her voice. Susan, in Chapter 10, writes to experience freedom of expression, as her husband serves time in a prison. In Chapter 11, Nancy, debilitated from multiple sclerosis, writes to empower herself. In Chapter 12, a young man writes to explore identity issues and combat mood swings. And, last of all, in Chapter 13, an eighty-year-old writes to review her life and the missing pieces of the jig-saw puzzle. Writing is a multi-dimensional tool, serving each person in a unique way.

Although we can never completely know the feelings of another person, these stories provide a portal to another human being's experience. The written lines form a web that sustains our human connection to each other. Your empathy and imagination are the passports. Through this portal, you will experience, in some small way, what it is like to be a soldier after battle, a teenager who becomes pregnant, an elderly person coming to terms with her final years, and other very real people.

These stories are filled with intense life challenges, so if you find yourself becoming anxious, please remember to exhale and take a break before you resume reading. It is impossible to encounter demons, or life challenges, without stress. It is difficult, even as an empathic reader, to witness these struggles without a quiver of strong emotion or an occasional lump in the throat. You will recognize the ten tranformative elements as you read each story. And it is possible that you may capture glimpses of your own story in the ones that follow.

~ 1 ~

The Woman Who Plowed Verses

Linda Lanza

According to the philosopher Rousseau, the basic necessities of life are air, water, and food.[1] For an artist, however, it is necessary to add one more element—impression. If every action has an equal and opposite reaction, the natural response to impression is expression. "One must give back the stare of the universe," writer Hortense Calisher once said.[2] The mind's eye is like an everpresent camera, constantly recording everything it sees. For artist Linda Lanza, these impressions serve as a source of creativity and self-knowledge.

As a calligrapher, Linda has studied the ancient Greek method of inscribing in which lines are written alternately from left to right. The Latin origins of the word "verse" describe a turning in lines or rows.[3] The Irish poet Seamus Heaney has compared this turning to the excavation of words plowing up from the unconscious.[4]

The following chapter traces an artist's response to a love relationship that ultimately threatens to destroy her. It is the story of a woman who plows verses, who diligently works to harvest what she believes her relationship can yield. It is a love story. It is also a story about the effects of alcoholism. This is Linda's story.

I AM A WORD PAINTER, a calligrapher. I make part of my living turning thoughts and feelings into tangible, enduring written forms. A good calligrapher uses the whole body to write. Like a farmer plowing, I lean in, the movement of my body inextricably woven to my breath. Sometimes emotions are so powerful that they cannot be totally contained in the body. When I harvest my emotional energy on paper, it is out of my body and someplace else. My handwritten journals seem to vibrate with the energy put into them.

One of the most challenging periods of my life was my relationship of sixteen years with a man who was an alcoholic. During that time I wrote my way through deceit, fear, and violence, both physical and emotional.

THE EARLY YEARS

Writing has always been my favorite toy and most magical source of entertainment. My fascination began as a toddler. I squirreled away my mother's discarded grocery lists and tried to replicate the shapes I saw there. When my father noticed how I played at writing, he decided to teach me for real. He was a poet and left-handed like me. Not surprisingly, I knew how to write before I entered school.

I was a child who lived inside my head. Worlds appeared before my inner eyes. I grew up in northwest Pennsylvania and northeast Ohio in a series of rural communities that tracked inland from Lake Erie. It did not matter to me that I had few friends; nature was my greatest constant companion. I was enchanted with my universe. I could sit for hours pulling apart a lilac leaf to see the skeleton veins. I wondered about the purpose of the beads on the backside of leaves or what caused the rain. My mother didn't like to answer questions and wasn't interested in things of the mind. Her lack of answers sent me to books, where I found a world of words that lit up my interior world. That is where I lived—in an interior world filled with lines, colors, and images.

In Mrs. Miller's first grade class, we all got newly sharpened pencils, tablets with dotted blue lines, and a pack of crayons. It felt like Christmas to me. I felt such reverence for these things that I memorized the order of the crayons so I could preserve my treasures: purple, green, orange, yellow, brown, red, black, and blue. I remember the rush I felt from the smell of the new books and fresh ink! It was hypnotic. I studied hard and was a serious student.

STABILITY IN CHAOS

My father was an alcoholic. He was a born writer, but made his living with his hands. He did roofing, heating, plumbing, working several jobs at once, always scheming to make ends meet for a family that grew to five children. Nearly every Saturday night there was a party at home that always involved a lot of drinking. The fun and dancing and silliness often turned mean. My father would seem to break out of his skin and fill the room. Emotions escalated. Frequently the yelling poured out into the street. Mom tried to calm him down: "George! George, come inside." I would comfort him, too. Dad treated me as though I were his parent, rather than his daughter. He expected me to understand more than I did. I adored my father and would do anything for him. It would be many years before I understood how his alcoholism affected all of us and some of the choices I made.

The drinking episodes became more violent with the years. Every holiday and birthday celebration was an excuse for mayhem. I remember one Christmas when I was eight. I was thrilled to receive a wooden highchair for my doll. By the end of the day, in a fit of drunken anger, my father had smashed it against the dining room wall into smithereens. What I had gotten that morning as a gift disintegrated before my eyes.

The learned expectation of incidents like this and more taught me early on that everything was transient. At least once a year my father moved us to a new town, or a different house in the same town, greener pastures while Dad tried yet another new thing to make a living. My brothers, sisters, and I had to leave behind what we couldn't carry or wouldn't fit in the next place. I was constantly in a new school and meeting new people, which was difficult for a child who was naturally shy and introspective. Consequently, the more I had to let go of people, the less attached I became to things and people, including myself, my own sense of myself.

Having been brought up in the Presbyterian faith, I believed the only way to be happy is to be of service to another. Having lived with constant insecurity, I had formed a habit of dependence. I began to feel like a cipher, someone without any kind of fixed identity or value except for how I could be useful to someone else.

Whenever my father discovered a talent of mine, he exploited it to the fullest. I started a typing course in tenth grade and within two weeks he had me in his office typing up marketing letters one by one. I didn't have the proper form down yet, or even know what to say, but he didn't care. He dictated the words and I typed them. Quantity was more important than quality to this man who had been orphaned at eight and grown up during the Depression. He walked me to the refrigerator once and opened the door. "Look at this! We're rich!" he said, gesturing to the food.

When I was fourteen, I asked for and received a guitar for Christmas. I had a good voice and had sung in my school choirs since the fourth grade. Before I knew it, my father had me accompanying him to bars in the evenings, propping me on bar stools and passing the hat around. I was a quick study. I listened to songs on the radio, took down the lyrics in short-hand, and figured out the chords by ear. Soon I was strumming out tunes by Peter, Paul and Mary, Tom Paxton, Buffy St. Marie, and Joni Mitchell. The things I couldn't say, I sang. I walked everywhere and gathered impressions that sprung to life on paper in collages, words, images, and songs.

I found I could protect my heart if I put it into a journal or writing. Writing was something no one could take away from me. The writer H.L. Mencken once wrote, "There's always a sheet of paper. There's always a pen. There's always a way out."[5] I didn't have to leave my journal behind. I took it with me wherever I went. I required little sleep. I often sleepwalked. Who knows? Perhaps I even journaled in my sleep. My mind and hands rarely stopped talking; my pen was never very far out of reach.

I left college after two years to move to Las Vegas and marry a man

I loved. I studied, practiced, and became a professional calligrapher and made part of my living teaching, writing wine lists, menus, and invitations, and working in situ to fill in participation certificates at the myriad conventions that frequented the city.

Single again in 1985 and still living in Nevada, I was attending an international calligraphy conference in California when I met Al. His sonorous voice, beautiful hands, and constant attention captivated me. I fell in love. Little did I know that his presence in my life would eventually turn to shadow and vapor.

> . . . *Some surprises sing you*
> *crystal clear soliloquies.*
> *Others will uproot you,*
> *discard you to your knees.*
>
> *Some will make you think you*
> *have the sky within your hand.*
> *Some surprises shake you*
> *like an hourglass full of sand.*
>
> *Some will make you blossom*
> *like rosebuds opening wide.*
> *Some surprises slash you,*
> *let heartbreak crawl inside.*
>
> *Some surprises take you*
> *where you think you might belong,*
> *but no surprises ache you*
> *like the one when love goes wrong.*

THE ENCHANTMENT

After four years of being single, Al looked very good to me. A wiry-built man in his forties, he was attractive and seemingly physically fit. He boasted a twenty-nine-inch waist of which he was quite proud. He had an extraordinary mind, and a witty sense of humor. We could see irony and absurdity in the same things. We were both visual artists who had majored in English in college. We loved the written word and shared a love of story. After the conference, I returned to Nevada and he went back to his home in New Jersey. We instantly began a written correspondence and daily phone calls. It was all poetry and magic.

I wrote about the wildflowers that peppered Red Rock Canyon, my children, my work, and music. He wrote about the East Coast, his work, his daughter, and music. He assured me he was divorced, and described in great detail his studio with a skylight. Photographs and magazine articles were exchanged. We visited each other's home. Words flew back and forth. When he asked me to marry him, I left Nevada and moved to be with him in New Jersey.

A WEB OF LIES

He deceived me from the beginning. Yes, I was gullible. I was lonely and hungry for some intimate personal attention. Al was a magnificent, well-practiced liar, and I must confess that I wanted to believe everything he said. I allowed him all the power of the decision-making. And yes, I would have bought the Brooklyn Bridge from him. But I would rather be the one who bought it than the one who sold it. There were little lies and big lies, but most of the lies were created to present a false self. He was not what he appeared to be—a healthy, creative artist who was a bachelor. In reality, he was a married alcoholic whose work life was rapidly spiraling downward from inattention and irresponsibility. He kept his twenty-nine-inch waist by drinking and hardly ever eating. He lived on sugared coffee and straight-up gin which he bought in the jumbo size twice or three times a week and stored behind his workbench, and which he drank from first thing in the morning to the last thing at night.

It was not his wife that concerned me. They had been leading separate lives for some time. It was his mistress that I could not compete with. She lived in a bottle and never left his side.

Mistress
translucent,
lustrous—her
luminous,
fiery jolt
is stronger.
She knows how
to bring you
back to her
every time.
No jasmine
water, no
diaphanous
drape, no wit
or laughter
does she give
to pleasure.
Only her
existence
is required,
enticing
forever.
Dress her in
familiar
crystal glass,
the family
heirloom, with
clinking ice—
four, five small
cubes—to suit

your mood, the
sparkling jewel
beckons. You
respond, en-
tranced by
your snow queen.
I turn my
back, tight fists
clutch blankets
to my neck,
as you kiss
her once more,
mesmerized,
before turn-
ing out the
bedroom light.

We had separate studios and worked at home. Al was remarkably good at the charade of being sober. I was often astonished to see him go from a staring stupor to an animated, lucid conversation when a business call came in. Then he would fall back into the trance after he hung up. He seemed to be able to turn it on and off at will in certain situations. You would think I would have gotten the picture a little sooner, say, at the conference where we first met. During one of the evening socials, Al had invited me to his room to show me his calligraphy kit. Among his brushes, paints, charcoals, and chalks was a Tangueray bottle of gin.

I recall the flash of recognition, that way alcohol has of sparking in me remembrances of the rousing carnival of family life my father and mother raised me in and which, in my mind, is some combination of catastrophe and safety in one picture. Not only did my notice of Al's gin bottle not stop me from going ahead with the intrigue of his romance, it pulled me forward toward something familiar and comforting; the good things that I had been exposed to as a kid outweighing (denying!) the chaos and mayhem that came with my alcoholic parent, so that the memory association was captivating. He felt like home to me.

There was much laughter early on, and a torrid sexual attraction that sustained itself through the years. But he was already hooked on alcohol when I met him, and alcohol was the driving force in his life.

The Internet and professional journals are peppered with credible research from the likes of the National Institute of Health on the effects of alcohol abuse, and its incurable, uncontrollable extreme, alcoholism, on the alcoholic and on those who live with and love them. Alcohol takes over the major systems and organs in the body. New cell growth slows and ceases. Any medicinal aspects of the distillation or infusion cease to be therapeutic and become toxic to the point of fatal. The brain actually shrinks in size. Whole lives are consumed.

Several times I poured Al's gin down the toilet, down the cellar stairs, out in the backyard in fits of frustration that became more and more frequent. Once I physically dragged him from the house to the car and drove him to our family doctor. The doctor arranged for a counselor from a rehab center to come to his office and meet with us. The counselor insisted we not even return home but go straight to rehab. Al would have none of it. He drew up inside himself and refused. In another episode, the doctor kept him in his office and gave him transfusions to treat dehydration. Al drank gin, not water, when he was thirsty. Finally the doctor gave Al the ultimatum that if he didn't stop drinking he would refuse to see or treat him.

I sought advice and assistance from Al's brother Joe. Many times he made the trip to our house to see how he could help. Always, Al turned off the stupor and turned on the big-brother charm so that it appeared that I was crazy for thinking there was anything wrong.

Several times I left Al and went back after each seductive assurance from him. I repeated this cycle several times. I had made a commitment. I felt torn in pieces. I was convinced that just one more thing would work, just one more step or moment or look or attempt or phone call or drop of water somewhere would turn the tide and all would be well with us finally.

Inertia

I fear, I think,
the discipline.
I fight, I think,
the restraint. I,
I fight, I think.
I fear, I think,
the fight. I fear
the fight. I fight
the fear, I think.

On Remote Control

Al insisted on photocopying my work. He became brooding and silent when I sold pieces or had work published. At first I took this as the highest compliment thinking that he wanted to keep them for himself rather than have me sell them. But calligraphy was how I paid my bills. Over time I realized he was using me. He needed to appropriate my work. To him there was no separation between my work and me, and his vantage point was that everything was his: his house, his garden, his car, his work, his family, his depression, his yard that needed mowing, his run of bad luck, his denial of an alcohol problem. My role was in-relation-to and as-quickly-as-possible. I was someone he could talk about socially. She this, she that, she cooks, she cleans, she paints, she irons, she dances, she does everything I want her to. He teased that he wished he had a remote control for me so he could just push a button and I would do whatever he wanted. I began to feel like a strip mine he quarried to garner social points.

When the demand for his style of hand-painted signage was usurped by computers, Al was unwilling or unable to adapt. People were no longer coming to him with commissions. His work needed marketing. Sometimes I lost work, pushing his art instead of my own. I made appointments for him, many of which he never kept. I learned the computer, but Al made no attempt to because he didn't have to. He had me. I cooked, did the laundry, kept the house clean, handled my business, helped with his business, and sometimes additionally worked 9-5 office gigs through a temp agency. I started back to college with a night class here and there to complete a degree that I hoped would increase my work prospects. Exhausted, I would come home and the lights would always be out. Al would be asleep or feigning sleep. His ever-present non-presence felt like a punishment. I couldn't understand how I could be working so hard yet be mired in debt with no light visible at the end of the tunnel, and with no shoulder to lean on albeit a man in my bed. And what exactly did he do all day while I was out working?

This poem, "Dimmer Switch," foreshadows the suspicion that I was giving too much and getting too little and that something had to change.

Dimmer Switch
Lights kept low—
dimmer switch,
round, plastic,
rotate to
adjust the
atmosphere,
—speak of fear
to give, beam
too brightly,
nothing to
give? Fear to
give wrongly?
Is giving
right, in any
case? Like grace?
Lights are up,
fearlessly.
Anyone home?

From within my ingrained dependence, I believed my security and happiness depended on my being useful, full of use. From inside the grip of his alcoholism, Al needed to use me to the point of abuse. We were classic co-dependents. Despite this seed of knowledge that was beginning to grow inside me, I continued to allow my life to be taken over by Al. He was a tyrant with the threat of violence just below the surface. I could feel it bubbling sometimes. Like my father, he ruled the roost. He had the final say about how and where we lived, what things we bought, who was allowed to visit, what we did for holidays, what was hung on the walls, and where each piece of furniture went. I wanted to please him yet be a person in my own right. Why did I want his approval, just as I had hungered for my father's? What was this demon: approval at any cost? Meanwhile, I was losing myself. One part of the self was watching the fragmentation take place:

More Real Than Apparent
I discard me like
reptiles shed skin. I wish I
didn't have to watch.

I needed to be desired and needed. Al needed to find out what I desired and needed so he could continue to withhold it from me as his way of wielding control in the myth of our relationship. He couldn't control his addiction, so he needed to control me. As I did more and more to try to gain his approval and have my needs met, I felt myself being pulled farther and farther into the recesses of myself for self protection, a familiar response to a familiar scenario. I began to have panic attacks and trouble breathing.

Although Al discussed our private business with other people, ironically he rarely said a word to me at home. In private, as the years and the alcoholism progressed, he did not engage me in conversations, did not compliment me for a meal well-made, did not ask my opinion about anything, did not respond to my questions with anything of substance that could resolve a matter, did not offer to take me anywhere away privately where we might refresh and renew ourselves together, did not speak my name to me.

Al became skilled at finding out what I needed and wanted and then withholding. He was trained as a spy in the Army during the Vietnam War. He filtered my phone calls from family and clients while I was out and did not relay messages. Years after the fact I learned of this. One repeat client searched for me for two years. He told me he had left five messages with my husband. I never received one. I wondered in that moment how many other messages, and from whom, I had never received.

SOUL LOSS

In the last few years of our relationship, Al's drinking became violent. My father had beaten the tar out of me more than once when he was drunk. Nevertheless, I was stunned and startled when, a few days after I received a $2,000 commission, Al beat me so badly I could hardly walk. In fighting back, I hurt my writing hand so badly I could barely hold a pen to work. Bruises and a black eye were a source of embarrassment. I hid for days at a time. I wanted to leave, and yet he begged me to stay. I left; he persuaded me to come back. I was afraid to leave, but I was reaching the place inside myself that said I was in worse danger if I stayed. I was losing my soul. An excerpt from a longer poem called "Cat Dance" captures the push-pull of our physical relationship after the night he beat me with his fists:

Cat Dance
. . . Now he was sitting on the edge of the coffee table,
the low, boxy construction he'd built from pressed
board planks, Formica veneer. He watched her.
I'm leaving, she murmured to the floor. Her shoulder

muscles charged and tightened. She inhaled deeply,
sat up straight, hands cupped palms up in her lap.
Her green eyes stared at the middle distance beyond him.
Whaddaya mean? He leaned forward, his gaze steady
on her, the whites of his eyes sharpening. A sunflower petal

floated to the floor. His eyes darted to it. I'm leaving,
she repeated, looking at him until he looked at her.
I've been gone a long time in my mind, and now

I'm going to get in the car and go.
Leaning back, he held her with his eyes.
The air thinned and whirled between
them. He sprung like a panther into her

lap. She fell backward against the sofa.
With both hands, in one motion, he ripped her
nightshirt up over her head, her panties down
her thighs and off. Instantly, his head was buried

between her breasts, now a breast in his mouth,
sucking now, his teeth gripping, his arms gasketed
around her, his hands clawed and grasped at her back.
Now his knees pried hers open. His hand under her

knee wrapped the leg it was a part of around
his waist. Now his hand pulled her hair, forced
her head back, exposed her neck. His mouth nipped
wildly at each invisible crevice. Now his hands

kneaded her, dragged her up against the armrest.
Her head dangled over it, arms untangled. His hands
pushed her knees up and open, hands wrapped her
legs over his shoulders like a fine, familiar coat,

and he, thrusting himself into her, danced
his wild cat dance.   They lay in a layer
as the rhythm of their breathing slowed and quieted.
He peeled himself away from her. He tried to stand up.
He sat down against the armrest. You know I

don't want you to go, he whispered from a dark pit
that opened somewhere near his stomach.
Unsure his spent arms would be able to hold it,

he plucked a petal, held it in his hand.
He stared at the velvety yellow wisp floating
in the sea of his palm. Yes. She
inhaled, audibly, like music. She opened

her eyes. Her twisted pile of limbs reformed
into a woman. She sat up, stroked the dark hair
on his forearm back and forth, back and forth. She plucked
the sunflower petal from his palm, brought it to her lips.

Yet I stayed. I couldn't believe that I could be working so hard and be participating so completely and fully in my life and at the same time be so miserable. I couldn't see a different way yet. I was imploding. "I'll do it" was an old, familiar mantra, a throwback to the days of exploitation by my father. I had picked a man just like Dad, and I was letting him destroy my life.

I found a way for me to raise my voice and state my case without screaming. The poetic form called anaphora (from the Greek "carrying back") is the repetition of the same word or group of words at the beginning of several consecutive verses. With repetition, the chant tends to build in emotional intensity. "That I'm Not" was a statement of resistance and a subtle declaration that my loyalty was coming to an end. I was not yet declaring who I was. First I needed to define who I was not.

War Weary Patriot Plots Treason

. . . that I'm not: the butcher,
the baker, the physician
to heal you, the madonna
to kneel you, the whore
to feel you, the cook

to meal you, the shyster
to deal you, the plastic
to seal you, the
light to real you;

. . . that I'm not: laugh lines
on your face, high-
octane fuel in your system,
salve for your war wounds—
battle scars, bumper cars,
empty jars, invisible stars;

that I'm not: attitude, platitude, Yo
dude, Quaalude, test tube, ruby,
amethyst, alexandrite sparkling away
the dark, the off, the down, the un-,
the non-, the yeah-but, the no-but,
the worst of it all that gains
confirmation, ratification, validation
in considered opinion (that I am not);

that I'm not: the man you didn't
become, the things you never did,
the things you don't possess, the places
you've never been, the joy
you do without, the shout,
the pout, time out!

that I'm not: the Masters degree,
the pedigree, the third degree,
the leisure spree, the magnolia
tree (let me be), the war debris,
the dynasty, just me,

equipped and empty
handed, palms up.

RAGE

It had been seven years or so into our relationship that I came to realize there was a serious contradiction between what I wanted and needed and what I was getting in the relationship. A few more years passed before I began to seriously wonder how uncanny it was that Al seemed always to pick up on my thoughts and mention exactly what was on my mind. I had thought of it as our "psychic connection." I finally realized that Al had a secret source. It was my journal.

One morning at the breakfast table he said something that was nearly a direct quote of what I had just written during my morning write in my journal. The betrayal I felt in that moment was so vicious that I feared I would become hysterical. I controlled my response with all my might as I looked at him with a frozen face. Years of loose puzzle pieces and small bewilderments came together in a picture that made me sick: he had been reading my journals all those years. As with gin and cigarettes, his sneaking into my journal became another addiction. I was one less thing to concern himself with if all he had to do was read my personal weather report in my journal. How easy he made it for himself.

Anger raged inside me, and I feared its destructive power. I was determined to deal with it in a constructive way. Inspired by the Greek concept of *temenos*, or sacred vessel, I chose a fine sheet of rag paper to act as a container into which I could pour these extreme feelings. I gathered a collection of quotations about anger. When I needed to vent, I went to the paper, spread it on my drafting table, and used whatever tools and media came to my hand without thinking about it. I focused on just staying with the emotion, channeling it onto and into the paper vessel. In the first three sittings, I was able to manage the anger through a process of concentrating my eyes on the paper, choosing tools, noticing each motion of diluted ink or gouache, and attending to my breath. On four separate occasions I raged on the page like Mount Vesuvius with the lava of hot anger pouring forth.

On the fourth occasion, my anger was so intense that I was out of control. I went to the paper, and try as I might to breathe and focus, my body got away from me. I stabbed at the page with my brush, and without any fore-thought wrote "She is Raging". As I stabbed the brush onto the paper I began to breathe more quietly. The tension in my body was gone. The anger was out and over. Not only was the paper a container for my emotional tidal waves, each mark was.

Al used my private streams of consciousness out of context and as his proprietary and primary way of interacting with me. While I was shower-ing in the mornings, Al had been reading my journals. For years. This real-ization concretized a turning point for me. It was the first time that I became consciously aware that I had to leave the relationship and change my cir-cumstances. My resentment grew as I began to realize that my trust and my strength had been and were being used against me and taken advantage of:

Use Tax I

Use my truths
against me?
Use my trust
against me?
Use my strength
against me?
Permission
is neither
asked for nor
granted.

CHOOSING LIFE

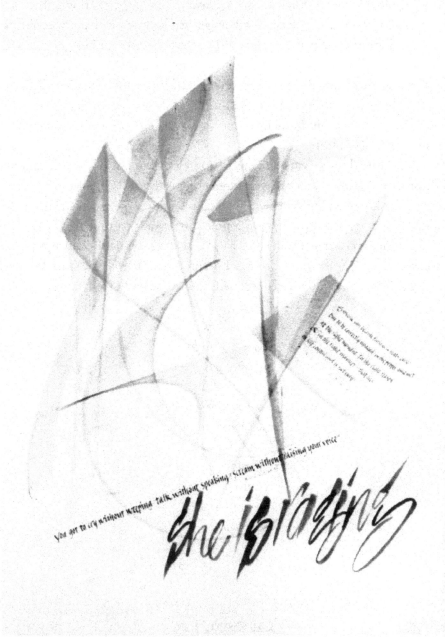

You got to cry without weeping, talk without speaking, scream without raising your voice

she is raging

Not long after this revelation, I took specific steps to leave the relationship for good. All traces of my trust and faith in him were gone. Moreover, I believed Al was consciously committing suicide with alcohol poisoning. I was not going to watch him do it, and I was not going to die with him. I came to realize that there was nothing more I could or would do for him. I chose life. I rented a small apartment near the Rutgers University campus and threw myself into studies in English to finish a degree.

Au Courant
Weathering white current,
red leaf abruptly
departs from the river.

Three years after I left Al, I got a call from the local police. An officer told me that Al had called her to say his wife was having trouble breathing and to send an ambulance. They responded immediately, but when they arrived at the house, there was no woman there, just Al in his underwear. I suppose they wondered where the body was, so they called me. I had to explain that yes, at one time I did have trouble breathing and had gone to the emergency room—about seven years earlier. I explained that Al had probably gotten confused about the memory because he had a drinking problem. "We know," the officer said.

Al's drinking had become such a concern to his brother that he had taken the battery out of Al's car, so he couldn't drive; instead Al called taxis to take him to the liquor store. He weighed less than 100 pounds when he died at age fifty-seven.

I had difficulty sleeping for about a year. My withdrawal from Al and the person I was when I was with him was a roller coaster ride of emotional adjustment comparable to narcotic withdrawal. His impressions on me ran deep. I had to learn how to trust again, and who. I had to learn new ways of feeling. Still I am learning.

Linda writes, "My withdrawal from Al and the person I was when I
was with him was a roller coaster ride of emotional adjustment compara-

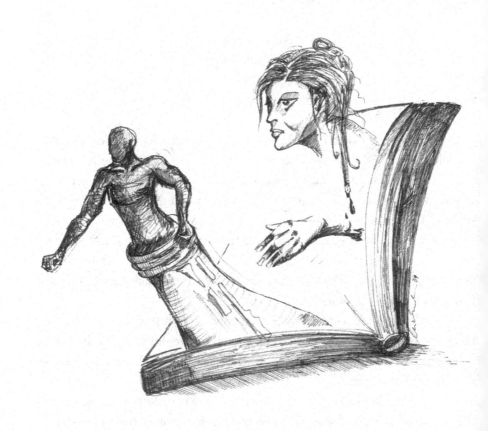

ble to narcotic withdrawal." Every dependent personality seeks a co-dependent.[6] If alcohol was Al's drug of choice, love provided the heady intoxication that Linda craved. And if every action has an equal and opposite reaction, just as Al was a master of control, Linda's life experiences had taught her to please and be as useful as possible. She astutely acknowledges her vulnerability when she writes, "Having lived with constant insecurity, I had formed a habit of dependence. I began to feel like a cipher, someone without any kind of fixed identity or value except for how I could be useful to someone else."

At the beginning of her relationship with Al, Linda believes she is a person whose freedom, safety, and privacy are intact. In time, Linda comes to understand that Al's need to control is violating every aspect of her life—psychologically, socially, and professionally. All five freedoms, as defined by Virginia Satir, are jeopardized: 1. the right to see and hear what is, instead of what should be, was, or will be; 2. the right to say what one feels and thinks instead of what one should; 3. the right to feel what one feels instead of what one ought; 4. The right to ask for what one wants, rather than permission, and 5. the right to take risks instead of choosing to remain secure and not rock the boat.

Linda discovers, with indisputable evidence, that Al has stolen her words, thoughts, and feelings by appropriating her journal. In a stunning epiphany, she realizes that his relationship to her is based on routine plundering. At that moment, she knows unequivocally that the relationship is over. At this point, her survivor instinct kicks in; she understands that she needs to leave if she wants to live.

Why did Linda stay in this relationship so long? First of all, Linda's ideas about love, commitment, and tolerance are in direct conflict with her growing recognition of abuse, creating an unbearable tension. Secondly, Al's violations are insidious and are not as apparent as the physical violence that is evident in "Cat Dance," when his alcoholism had progressed.

Meanwhile, Linda's "inner camera" records her images, thoughts, and feelings. These impressions are vital to her existence. By reading and reflecting on her own words, Linda is able to witness her own frustration, fear, and rage, as well as her desire to make this relationship work at all costs.

Linda's journal reflects four important therapeutic dimensions of writing: 1) writing for organization and clarification; 2) writing for catharsis and self-regulation of emotion; 3) writing for reflection; and 4) writing for problem-solving. All four functions provide the writer with a sense of empowerment and mastery. Linda's rite of journal writing is a way for her to stay in touch with a rich and emotional inner landscape. Initially, the journal acts as a magnetized catcher's mitt, a container to collect, organize, and integrate all the impressions, thoughts, and feelings into one unfragmented whole. Secondly, Linda strives to be emotionally balanced through the containment and release of excess emotions. "War Weary Patriot Plots Treason" and the calligraphic rendering of "She is Raging" are powerful examples of expressive, cathartic writing. When the writings are re-read, clarification and reflection take place. This function is evident in "Use Tax I," with the words, "Use my strength against me? / Permission is neither / asked for nor / granted." It is also demonstrated in the observations voiced in "More Real Than Apparent": "I discard me like / reptiles shed skin / I wish I / didn't have to watch."

Problem-solving, the fourth therapeutic dimension, is sometimes a slow process. Years pass between the writing of "Mistress," a poem in which Linda clearly recognizes the enticing "other woman" in Al's life, and "Au Courant," in which a red leaf abruptly departs from the river. In truth, Linda's leaving is not sudden. Each day moves her slowly towards taking a step that is excruciatingly difficult.

Caught between her need to love and be loved, and her need to be her own person, Linda goes back and forth as she struggles in this difficult relationship. This "plowing" is hard work; it is a daily process of turning thoughts and feelings over until the fertile earth is ready for new seeds of life. Word-flowers rise up from the fertile swampland of the subconscious into consciousness. When Linda learns that which she *already knows—after much twisting and turning—the woman who plows verses finds her true direction.*

~ 2 ~

The Poem That Was
Snake Medicine

Preston H. Hood, III

*Preston is a Vietnam Veteran. His journey of healing from Vietnam
began in 1970 and continues into the present. It is his realization that war
is a serpent that eats its way inside you and alters you forever. In almost
every poem that he has written about the war, there is the presence of a
snake or the sound of a rattle. The snake symbolizes the insidious and poi-
sonous effects of war.*

*Veterans and other survivors of trauma are subject to a group of
symptoms that we call post-traumatic stress disorder (PTSD).[1] This is
a condition of persistent stress caused by exposure to a life-threatening
situation. Typically there is sleep disturbance and frequent vivid recall
of the traumatic experience. There are dulled responses to others and
to the outside world; much psychic energy is used to keep painful memories from reaching awareness. Flashbacks are shocking images that the
brain was not able to process at the time of the trauma. These memories are released slowly over time.*

Preston began writing seriously when he was in Vietnam. He worked and reworked the same poem for over twenty-five years. He wanted to be truthful to the images that he had seen. At the same time, his mind was struggling to recall and integrate all he had experienced. Writing was a way to re-member the story in order to become whole again.

This is Preston's story.

THE EARLY YEARS

My childhood had the stability of a jumping bean—going off in different directions at the same time. My mother was an alcoholic, so, when I was born in 1943, I spent my first eight weeks in an incubator. My identical twin brother died at birth. I can only wonder who he would have been in my life. My father was a successful lawyer and later a lieutenant commander in the navy, but as a father there is only one word to describe him—absent. He spent as little time as possible with the family. He did not want to be around my mother because he didn't understand her, and since I was the eldest of two other siblings, I tried my best to protect my sisters from my mother's alcoholic rages.

I felt alone, even though I had friends to play with. My greatest companion was my grandfather. He took me for long walks in the woods and showed me how to use a knife. Gramp introduced me to poetry. I still remember the words to Alfred Noyes' poem "The Highwayman" and Rudyard Kipling's poem "If" that we recited together. Gramp also was the person who taught me how to communicate and be a caring person. He was more a father to me than my father was.

I started writing humorous verse when I was a teen. When I wrote, I felt better. So I kept on writing. In my youth, writing was a way to help me laugh.

I wasn't much of a student. I couldn't be. I often didn't get much sleep at night. I would be awakened by my mother. At night she drank herself into a stupor, but before doing that, she would fall down the stairs to get my attention. She took me to the den to talk after my father left when they had an argument. My mother would yell and belittle me until four or five in the morning then she would pass out. At times she was sexually inappropriate and wanted me to fill in for my absent father. I was the awkward, confused custodian of the family. There was much I did not understand.

By the time I was eleven, I was one screwed up kid. I was always in trouble in school. I did crazy things. For example, one time in school, I smashed my fist into my nose and smudged the blood along the hall door window. Now I can recognize that as a cry for help, but back then, I acted out instinctively; it was my knee-jerk reaction to a world that didn't make much sense to me. I was aware that my father hoped I would become a lawyer like him and his father. In his fantasy the law office would read, "Hood, Hood, and Hood." Everything inside me said, "No, No, and No." It was a life I wanted no part of. I was not proud to be Preston Hood, III. I remember flunking out of high school. My parents sent me to a psychiatrist. I stood there in my argyle socks, corduroy pants, and cap, and when the psychiatrist asked my name, I said, "I'm Little Lord Corduroy." That is the only thing I would say. Within a few minutes, he gave up trying to get me to talk.

I was sent to boarding school, where I had a more normal existence, excelling in sports—football, track, and skiing. Although I had never touched a book in high school, at prep school I had a great English teacher who inspired me. I read a hundred books in two years. My college education was sporadic, and I did not complete my college degree at this time. After being kicked out of college a number of times, I found work as a laborer. I learned to be a mason's tender. For the time being I was happy doing this work. And then the draft came. I wanted no part of that, so in 1966 I joined the Navy like my father. Whatever demons I possessed from a difficult childhood paled in comparison to the demons that followed.

THE WAR

When I first joined the Navy, I went to basic training at Great Lakes, Illinois. Because I could scuba dive, they felt I would be valuable in underwater demolition teams. After my first duty station, I finally passed the qualifications for BUDS, Basic Underwater Demolition Seal training. It was a very grueling sixteen weeks. There were 139 of us beginning the training, and only seventeen men made it. There was a one-week period called "Hell Week" during which we were allowed a total of only three hours of sleep. They wanted to see how we would function under extreme conditions. The three hours were broken into ten- or fifteen-minute catnaps. Many men couldn't take the sleep deprivation, the drills that pushed our bodies to their limit, the harsh demands, and the psychological cruelty employed. They broke down and quit. At one point, I thought I had broken my ankle and was sent to sick bay for an x-ray. On my return, the instructors harassed me twice as much as before to see if I would quit. I had missed a training evolution, and the instructors definitely did not like that. They said to me, "Hood, you have a Cadillac body and a Volkswagen engine, you better keep up!" I did keep up and did not quit.

I was chosen to become a Navy Seal and was damn proud of it. By the time that training was complete I was invincible. I felt as if I could walk through a wall. I wanted to serve my country and now I had a way to do it. I never imagined what horrors would follow.

I was trained to be a killing machine. I never questioned it. I performed as I was trained to perform. The drills were repeated over and over— Never leave a man behind. And KILL. It is okay to kill. KILL, KILL, KILL— Have no mercy. KILL. Hurrarh!

I spent seven months in Vietnam. Little did I know then that these seven months would irrevocably shape the years that followed. Whatever I saw and endured went underground. For the first ten years back from Vietnam, I thought I was fine. But I had an exaggerated startle response to any noise, and I did not sleep well. When I did sleep, I would often wake in a cold sweat. I was also much quicker to anger than I had been before. Nevertheless, I led a normal life with the woman I married and was living off the land in Maine in a home I had built myself. We had a biological child and adopted two children and were raising them in a home without plumbing or electricity. It was a simple life but it was good one. Being near the land was healing for me.

Curiously, more than a decade passed before memories started to surface. I had flashbacks and would awake shaking and in a sweat and screaming. At home, my anger unleashed itself as I yelled at my wife and children. As the years went on, more memories came back and I anchored them to the page by writing them out. It was a way of trying to understand what had happened. The war had become a blur. I had very little recall of actual events. Memories came back to me, piece by piece, like a jig-saw puzzle.

I wrote only one poem when I was in Vietnam. In "Rung Sat" I tried to grasp the reality of this war. It was a collage of some of the experiences I had in Vietnam, and helped me to put things into perspective. It took me twenty-five years to rewrite this poem until I was finally satisfied. The poem is significant because it was the first time I was honest with myself about what I had done. The poem serves as a witness.

Rung Sat is a jungle where the North Vietnamese Army (NVA) and Viet Cong (VC) entered South Vietnam. The words "orange mist" refers to Agent Orange, a chemical defoliant sprayed in Vietnam. The substance is now widely believed to be carcinogenic, but its toxicity was not known by many veterans at the time. I suffered, as did many others, from sores and still have numbness and circulation problems. Our faces were camouflaged, but our hands and arms were exposed. The orange mist would float down, and we had no idea what it was. We didn't realize we would live with its after-effects all our lives.

Rung Sat

I rappel through the door of the gunship
thinking about someone to love.
On patrol I'm a hunter in the blackness
dozing off, hardened, tired of danger,
I sight the enemy, belly wet deep
in Rung Sat,
muscular legs standing executioner quiet,
black-green smudge and sweat curled on lip.
A snake stops me. I wade ahead,

fall through myself like a stone,
enemy voices passing only meters away,
the back drop of dark, life's death.
I scan the horizon for movement,
count the bodies across the canal,
wait until they slip into the mud.
My mind is a red-brown blur,
a gauze for the wounded we torture.
What's happening seems not true.

Two hours before dawn the next day, we insert
by chopper, on some Viet Cong farmer's land
to interrogate sympathizers,
and search for the mortar tubes
the NVA shell us with.

We demand revenge:
the smell of rice at the jungle top,
lazy orange mist shifting like smoke.

In low silhouette, we patrol to ambush—
our bodies surrounded by dark—
the shadow of surprise suspended inside us.
Across the trail, wind rips nipper palm,
fear crawling at our feet, like a wounded man.

We radio in an air strike—
the wounded lie with the dying,
the dragged bodies, hurried away
disappear into bamboo.
Blood trails along the river
mark a company retreat—
abandoned bombed-out bunkers

shallow graves dug quickly,
brown-uniformed and black pajama bodies,
rice bowls and fish heads—
children half-buried in dirt.

I am a man half in the water, half out;
my legs suck into mud.
My arms hold my head outstretched—
hasten to deliver me among the dead.

"I am a man half in the water, half out." This line captures the way I felt many years later—one foot in this world and one foot in the other. I felt numb and half-dead when I was in Vietnam. Part of me was almost begging them to kill me. Like John the Baptist, I wanted to be delivered. I was tormented by guilt, but not yet conscious of that. This poem and the others I wrote serve as witness and testament. They are the recordings of the stories that everyone wants to forget.

At one point I was shot in the leg and the stomach, and for six days lay in Bien Hoi third field hospital, while they drained my wounds. It was the first time I had time to think. I started to wonder, "What am I doing here?" I felt a heavy grief in my chest. In the hospital library, I read Keith Wilson's *Graves Registry* and *The Ugly American*. We were taught to hate the people; they were the enemy. I only questioned this when I was out of action. Guilt and grief slowly made their way to my consciousness over the next two decades. Thirty years later I wrote the following:

Grief Attaches Itself to My Chest (for my medic Sandy Lang)

i
Like a leech it sucks me cold.
Like a snake it eats its way
inside me
sheds its skin;
its sadness
becoming me, becoming him

48

a rage of two minds split
  an ache so deep inside
I say fuck it,
    fuck it to all.
Fuck the undone war
    the carpet bombing
the men we left behind.
    Fuck all the people
all the planners of that war.

ii

In nightmares I thought I left behind
    I'm lost,
searching for prayer,
and the missing heads of brothers.

iii

I awake in an abandoned village,
    the devil licking his tongue,
a love I was unable to have,
    I was unable to touch.
The serpent worm bores
    through my body.
I hate the sleepless nights on the ward
    the wasted days, the grief
circling above my heart.
    I leave one place for another,
and never arrive.

I was in Vietnam for seven months, but it seemed like forever. For the Vietnamese people who had fought the French, China, the United States, and Pol-Pot in Cambodia for decades, war really was endless. Women and men chew on "betel nut juice" to get high. There are few pleasures and no security. People are surviving, not living. Imagine being at war your entire life.

Ho Chi Minh City

Imagine a square of whiskey odor
near a jaundiced river
where girls in ao dai zip

into the darkness on Hondas,

nipper palm yellows in dry heat
and an old woman squatting spits

betel nut juice into the street:
imagine being at war
for your entire life.

Note: Ho Chi Minh City is the new name given to Saigon, Vietnam, after the North won the American war. Ao dai (pronounced ow zi) is a traditional dress worn by Vietnamese women.

AFTER THE WAR

When I came home, I was silent and numb. Soldiers returned from Vietnam, not as heroes but as despised men. I was spit on upon my return and called a "baby killer." There was no glory, no hero's triumph. We were hated by most, tolerated by some. To many people, Vietnam was a mistake, a war that should never have taken place. Attitudes of our fellow Americans shamed us and served to further insure our silence and slow our recovery. Whatever memories surfaced would do so "under cover," in our nightmares, our flashbacks, and our states of reverie.

In the next poem, I ask, "What heart will find them (the soldiers) worthy of love?" In other words, "Who will love us?" We were hated by the enemy, but far worse than that, we were despised by our own people. It was hard not to feel that hatred; it was easy to turn it against oneself. The Christ images in the poem—the crown of thorns, the nails through my feet—suggest the sacrifice that was made by American soldiers.

Against Fear

Life ending could go like this:
slivers of shrapnel rip into the body—
pain cuts the imagination deep
the hollow of the brain shuts down—forever.
Why is fear a weeping eye, a crown of thorns?
Why am I convinced someone
is driving nails through my feet?

In the battlefield of hate
when I am a rabbit being eaten by a snake
what will happen to the thoughts of my men?
What will claim their miserable souls?
What high moment will stop them
from shrieking as they cross an open field?
What heart will find them worthy of love?
Within men's passion of triggers—the flash
which happens faster & slower & back again—
marches a world of non-violence.
Beneath the scar—the deep
incision in the souls of men—
is there a moment & a person
that may make all the difference to them?

In the first decade upon my return, I evaded my memories by keeping busy. In 1973 I completed my B.A. in English, Magna Cum Laude at the University of Massachusetts, Boston. After my degree, I left the "Do this, Do that" signs of the city for living off the land in Maine. I worked on the land, ran marathons, built my home, raised my kids and in 1983 got an Associate Degree in Applied Technology and Carpentry from Northern Maine Technical

College. I was a slow bloomer in education. But once I got started, I couldn't stop. That same year, I accepted a job as an industrial arts teacher and went on to get a B.S. in Industrial Arts Technology from the University of Southern Maine, in 1987. Ten years later, I was still going to school and working as a special education teacher when I attained my Masters Degree in Special Education Administration from the University of Maine, Orono, in 1997.

I can admit now that I was a workaholic. I just kept moving as fast as I could, hoping to outrun the memories. In the 1990s, I became an assistant principal and an athletic director and even that was not enough, so in 1997, after my graduation, I became a director of Special Education in New Hampshire. In 2000 we had about twenty bomb scares in the district where I supervised, and I was one of the staff who had to investigate what was really happening. During this time the flashbacks came back full force. My heart would race. In terror, I would break out in cold sweats. Time blackouts would occur. I would be in a bomb threat situation one minute, then back in Vietnam, and hours later I would be driving around in a car and suddenly realize I had no idea where I was. The flashbacks were vivid and painful. I started to recall people and events that my mind had blocked out. Terrible scenes of broken bodies and body parts haunted me. In addition, a suicide I had witnessed back in Vietnam, and had blocked out for thirty years, came back to haunt me. I wrote to anchor my ghosts. In another memory, I will never forget the young girl who approached with grenade in hand on one of our search and destroy missions.

Girl Blown Apart

That night is like a starlight scope
with weak batteries, fades
in and out. A night thick with heat.
Groping under the camouflage of our shadows.

We didn't care
beyond the river of blood
if we leveled the place, unleashing
ourselves like venomous snakes,

cutting throats for a body count.
On the way out, a very young
uniformed girl soldier,
raised her hand to throw grenades.

. . . the black wound of this memory
re-opens . . .
Monkeys calling. Rain
across Buddha's arms. Death's

rattle in my ears—my m-16
blew out her cheek. The war
continues to flank me, a black
horse. And her ghost

winters in the chunk
of my unkempt head where I can't
suture the gash between
sadness and death.

In the 1990s, I felt my life was unraveling. I was stressed out and exhausted. I couldn't run or work through it anymore. In 1995, my wife and I separated, and in 2000 we divorced. The same year, I resigned from my job due to flashbacks and stress. On one occasion, during a bomb sweep, I opened a package, wondering if a bomb might be inside. Suddenly, I found myself crouched on the ground next to my car, experiencing a flashback of the Vietnamese woman and two children who were killed by our rockets. I was still in a daze afterward and missed a very important court date for one of my students. I was suffering more PTSD symptoms than ever before.

Not only was I reliving the events during the day; I revisited them in my nightmares as well. It was affecting my work and my personal life. I was always on guard and was emotionally numb. I tried to avoid any situation that could trigger traumatic feelings. I would retreat into myself and would not talk. I couldn't sleep. I was always irritable and had difficulty concentrating. To make matters worse, my youngest son committed suicide when I entered the PTSD program. I was angry and depressed and didn't care if I lived or died.

RECOVERY

I knew I needed help. Fortunately, during this time, I heard about the North Hampton, Massachusetts, Veterans Administration Medical Center's PTSD Program. This program plays a pivotal role in my eventual rehabilitation. The sense of fraternity and compassion that the men of Ward 8 gave each other was and is very healing. Suddenly I realized that I wasn't alone. Amongst ourselves we shared in the Vietnam War experience; we all had experienced death and trauma in a very similar way. We all felt loss for our buddies; we felt guilt and all had severe startle response. We all shared endless, ever-present fear and anxiety. Because we experienced these things, we were very close to each other.

It was other people that we did not trust. Others did not understand what we had been through. However, the staff on Ward 8 did care, and for the first time we were treated with kindness, respect, and understanding. Eventually we learned to trust others. Every winter is especially difficult for me because the anniversary dates of some of the most horrendous patrols in Vietnam come back to me at this time. Every year I go back and renew the skills I learned from this program, because these skills help keep me focused so that I am able to move on with my life. The next poem is dedicated to all the veterans and staff of Ward Eight:

After Ward 8

I wake in a strange place,
    the window open,
a speeding train, I'm tired.
    No black coffee for days.
Snow falling, the open
    window of knives
wants absolution.
    End of April '01,
the snow has not yet melted
    nor has the ice on the lakes gone out.

Before the end of winter
    I'm a fallen stone, a stony heart.
I hear the rattle of the snake,
    my words on a deaf ear.
I enter the river of vertigo through my eyes:
    sands whirl, crows scatter.
The rescue takes longer, slower
    through the thunderheads and closed sky.
Drowned in voices, I lose myself
    like a dry seed
through a rain stick.
Light falls across wet lilacs
erases the years, careening
over everything.

I also participated in the Outward Bound Program, which was very helpful in my gaining back my self-esteem. This program was the last Veteran's Outward Bound Program to be held, and many of us hoped we would be chosen. Thirteen veterans were selected to participate in the program. I was very happy to be one of them. Some of the veterans were from our group, and others had previously gone through the PTSD program. The plan was to take us to the woods and have us go on a fifty-mile trip. Then we had to hike a mountain and rappel down the other side. We finished the program by teaming up with another vet and going through an obstacle course. The final night was a sweat lodge experience that was very personal and spiritual. Each one of us chose things we wanted to let go of and used the sweat lodge as a catalyst for the letting go. It was good to be in nature as it helped us all pull together and be ourselves for the first time in many years.

Little did we know that the next day, on our graduation, the events of 9/11 would take place. It would change our world as we knew it. Most of all, we were glad we were there together for this experience. The camaraderie we shared made it easier for each one of us to deal with the situation. What was even more special when we arrived back at the VA was the welcome home dinner we received from the veterans and staff at Ward 8. We finally got the well-deserved welcome home that we had never received before.

Another important workshop some veterans and others have attended was the William Joiner Center for War and Social Consequence's Writer's Workshop. In 1989, I attended my first writer's workshop along with my North Vietnamese counterpart. For the first time, each of us talked and wrote about our shared war experiences. We were not enemies now. We were trying to understand and be friends. How different was that!

The millennium ushered in a new era in my life. For almost thirty years, since the war, I had written only dark poetry. But now, I started to write more humorous poetry again. Before the war, writing was a way for me to laugh. After the war, it was a way for me to cry. But with the new millennium, I was a more complete and healthy person. Now I could laugh and cry in my writing and in my life. I met a wonderful woman, and we married. I chose a new life style that would reduce the stress in my life. I retired and went back to living near the earth in Maine. It is true that I still have my many moments with PTSD, but I don't have the symptoms as often. I am coping with my PTSD, but know that at any time it can ambush me in the shadows. Here is a poem I wrote about all of us moving together for peace.

Millenium of Hope

At the top of the mountain
looking back toward the East
I lean on memories like rifles
& watch the lanterns spilling light
onto the midnight of fear—

I look back over three decades
& see Vietnamese children
break down into tears, then
in fading fall light, a chill wind,
the heartache of Vietnam Veterans facing the Wall.

I see candles of hope,
a new millennium of truth
striving to prove that the self
is finally able to let go
of the updraft of war—
into thinnest air—
the imprinted image
at the fall of Saigon—
the clinging & falling
of ARVNS—that last liftship
take off from the embassy roof.

The full moon eclipses:
clouds fly between
the GI & VC gazing
into wildest light.
the distance between
then & now
becoming seamless.

At midnight there comes a rattling,
shadows move secretly
voices drift low
toward the river,
the South China sea
where another boat of humanity
pulls away with memories
of Nui Ba Den, Black Virgin Mountain.

The obvious demons of war are death, destruction, and hatred. But compliance and denial are also demons. We thought we could kill, and then put it aside, as though it were of no import. We thought America was about God, country, and apple pie, yet we made our young men into killing machines. And afterwards, it was just a mistake.

How have we been patient
all these years
struggling with pain & doubt
of naiveté to erase the war
from our hearts & minds
inching up to the millennium?

The pieces of the puzzle are finally coming together for me. Writing has helped me to reclaim my memories and become whole. My veteran brothers have given me support and have been my comrades. My wife, Barbara, has helped me to find laughter and joy again in life. And the rattling of the snake is getting more and more distant, but will always be there.

What Comes Next

We find the end by mixing tears with happiness
burning with the agony of how much war consumes
knowing no love or god or spirit can claim us
by revisiting all the paths we've walked, all the darkness
we traveled, the sorrow in the mouth deep love we lived.
We find the constellations of our lives by dismantling the pain

of the body, enduring the past of our delinquencies,
while recovering the lost youth stripped from us.

& in the earth forever time we see the life for what it is:
a hand that leads us, irrevocably, into sorrow
here, we desperately insist on passion
wandering among the dead of us, within
the old shells of our bodies wondering whether
something laughable or peaceful or real comes next.

Preston's poetry is his "snake medicine." The distant rattle of the snake reverberates through almost every poem. The Ouroboros is an ancient symbol depicting a serpent swallowing its own tail and forming a circle. It has many meanings—among them the cyclical nature of life and death, transformation, unity or wholeness, and infinity.[2] Psychologist Carl Jung believed that it had an archetypal significance in the human psyche, symbolizing the assimilation of the opposite, particularly significant to his theory of integrating the shadow self and individuation.

The snake brings forth a new self by shedding its old skin in a transformational process. The poems mirror the cognitive process that occurs in post-traumatic stress disorders. In a sense, each poem is a piece of snakeskin, released and outgrown. During Preston's flashbacks, time and space are shifted, as his memory unexpectedly takes him back to Vietnam. In a series of starts and stops, the brain downloads each image, often when Preston least expects it. In an act of mastery and creativity, Preston captures these images through the poetry. When Preston externalizes the images by converting them to ink, he can view the toxic images at a safe distance. He is also able to stand back to witness the experience with new understanding. When he captures the image to his satisfaction, he is empowered. When he edits and re-edits, he exercises artistic freedom and control of the process.

Rarely does a poem take twenty-five years to complete. However, it takes Preston twenty-five years to create "Rung Sat" because his mind has withheld certain information, holding significant images hostage for more than two decades. Only after these involuntary and terrifying images have been downloaded in entirety can the poem be completed. Its completion coincides with a time period of great chaos and transformation in his personal life—the shedding of marriage, job, and residence. Before Preston could lay claim to a happier and healthier life style, he needed to let go of the pain and rage that had accumulated from his losses in childhood, in Vietnam, and in a marriage that was filled with resentment. Preston then lays claim to a healthier, happier lifestyle, retiring in the country and writing his poems again.

Snake is representative of the life-death-rebirth cycle; similarly, Preston, with the support of loving friends and family, is able to regenerate (re-create) himself. He will always have his symptoms of PTSD, but in time he will hopefully gain some peace.

Snake energy, according to its mythology, is the energy of wholeness, cosmic consciousness, and the ability to experience anything willingly and without resistance. It teaches that all things are equal in creation. War is a direct violation of this principle. It is about fragmentation and destruction. Anyone who survives the fire of battle stares directly into the face of death, and literally endures "trial by fire."

Although Preston writes for the purpose of organization and self-regulation through containment and cathartically venting, his primary goal is the integration of his traumatic war memories. He writes to metabolize pain. Disturbing undigested images remain unprocessed in the revolving door of pain. Preston is downloading these images, converting them from his mind's eye into poetry, expanding the time in order to process the memories completely.

Poetic justice suggests that while war is an act of destruction, writing is, symbolically, an act of restitution and creativity. While trauma separates the person from the world, writing can also be a statement to return the victim to the world. Writing workshops for veterans such as the William Joiner Center for War and Social Consequence's Writer's Workshop have been very successful. By sharing among other veterans, the trauma is not borne alone. Preston has taken this one step further. By reading for the general public, Preston has moved the private trauma into the public arena, to be witnessed by all. He has courageously removed the taboo of silence that so many returning veterans observe.

War is alienating, destructive, and fragmenting; writing is unifying, integrative, and opposes silence. Writing is an underused transformational tool that may assist veterans in moving through the necessary process of articulating the trauma, witnessing, mourning, and integration.

It is said that poison can be ingested, and if one survives, it is possible to transmute the toxins. Preston is absorbing and integrating the poison, rendering it less toxic with each poem he writes. He is performing one of the most difficult of all transformations; the conversion of blood to ink![3]

~ 3 ~

Greetings from CancerLand
Alysa Cummings

As Nietzsche once said, "That which does not kill me makes me stronger."[1] There are about ten million men and women cancer survivors for whom Nietzsche's message resonates most powerfully.[2] Approximately one in eight women a year hear their doctors speak the terrifying words—"You have breast cancer."[3]

Following diagnosis, women make a survivor's journey through CancerLand, a path fraught with fear and uncertainty all along the way. On a psychological level, knowing that something toxic is growing wildly out of control inside of you, that your own body has betrayed you, that a tumor could in fact kill you, is the stuff of nightmares. How do breast cancer survivors manage to cope?

During the treatment phase many doctors in CancerLand keep their focus on the physical realm; the emotional dimension may be overlooked. For breast cancer survivor Alysa Cummings, journaling was a healing prescription she wrote for herself to spiritually recover from cancer treatment. Here is her story.

THE CANCERLAND JOURNAL

His name is Boris. He is trying to kill me. I won't let him.

And so my CancerLand journal began: with three short sentences, a stream of words that had been swirling around in my head for days, days that otherwise had been spent in and around the health care delivery system visiting assorted doctors (gynecologist, radiologist, breast surgeon, oncologist) for painful tests followed by frightening results. I remember endless crying jags and repeated phone calls to my insurance company. In my bedroom at night, I would stand in front of my full length mirror, my shirt hiked up high on one side, and stare at my upper body—shocked and wide eyed, hypnotized by my reflection, all the while muttering to myself, "So this is what cancer looks like. So this is what cancer feels like."

His name is Boris. He is trying to kill me . . . I repeated these words under my breath like a prayer, my very own disease mantra. Call it the ravings of the recently diagnosed, but the words helped me focus—on the next decision, the next appointment, the next step on the path. The words also kept me slightly sane, all things considered; imagine talking yourself down from the ledge. The words begged to be tapped out on a keyboard, so I followed the urge, liked how it made me feel in the moment and then just kept typing.

I hate Boris. Boris has been lurking in my chest for ten years possibly, hiding, madly multiplying, growing, only now choosing to make his obnoxious presence felt.

Who was Boris? (Yes, I confess that I named my tumor, personifying him as Boris Badunov of Rocky and Bullwinkle cartoon fame.) Writing about Boris and plotting his imminent demise helped me wrestle with my first real demon—that I had no control. Never had, never would. Over anything related to cancer, which by its very definition, means life out of control.

Boris. Foreign. Evil. Pint-sized. If I can picture my enemy I can fight him;

at the very least I can write about him. Am I writing for my life?

I fantasized that I could somehow use my computer to craft a story with an upbeat next chapter. Or a fairy tale, happily-ever-after ending even. Looking back, that's the only explanation I can come up with, why I felt so compelled to create a record of my day-to-day experiences as a cancer patient. The one thing I could control were these words that crowded each other as they quickly appeared on my computer screen; these stories that flowed through my fingertips in such a manic rush, these traumatic adventures that happened to me in a place I began to call CancerLand.

CancerLand: it's this parallel universe, I swear, separate and apart from the rest of life as I once knew it. How did I end up in this wacky Bizarro World filled with freaky language and even stranger rituals?

THE CANCERLAND JOURNEY BEGINS

It was late October 1998, and I remember being stretched out on my couch in the den watching the evening news. There was one of those predictable stories about Breast Cancer Awareness Month that ended with the reporter promoting monthly self-examination, and my hand moved with a mind of its own to my right breast. And that's when I felt it: a lump.

By Halloween, I was flat on my back on the gynecologist's examination table with a syringe sticking out of my chest.

The holes in the ceiling tiles shift crazily in and out of focus. Dots. Holes. Shadows. Connect the dots. I squeeze the nurse's hand much too tightly and wonder if all the sweat I feel is mine. I smell myself; my own sticky fear. I don't like it, the doctor says, finally removing the needle. It's very bloody. Not acting like a cyst at all. The bandage on my chest is a small square with a red circle in the middle. The flag of Japan, I think to myself. The doctor reassures with lots of nervous pats on my leg. Then the door slams and I am alone and shaking. I pull on my jeans and trash the paper gown. Something has changed. I know it. Feel it intuitively. For the first time I have seen cancer reflected in a doctor's eyes. It won't be the last.

The gynecologist's needle biopsy is inconclusive, so before week's end I have my first encounter with a breast surgeon.

This Breast Surgeon

They look at the films together.
Oh, I don't like this. I don't like this one bit, he says.
This breast surgeon points to her x-ray
Traces lazy circles with his fingertips
Reaches for a small white writing pad
(The name of a pharmaceutical company
Printed across the top) Starts drawing breasts.
He quickly creates a female torso
Just one unbroken line from his black felt tip marker.
A moment later a straight shorter line turns into an arm;
A curved half circle becomes a breast.
Another much smaller circle appears
Suddenly there's a nipple; then two: a matched set.
In a stupor of silent anxiety, she watches him sketch,
Thinks about Picasso; drawings so evocative
With one simple, continuous line.
And as she spectates, a soothing mantra
Spins through her head:
This man has sketched millions of breasts.
He is good at drawing breasts.
He is good at cutting breasts.
He knows breasts.
This breast surgeon.

Waiting for the breast surgeon's biopsy results is agonizing. Pretending that life is normal, business as usual. It's all an act. Going through the motions. But just ask any cancer survivor. There is a soul level sense of knowing the results even before the report lands on the doctor's desk. And then, of course, the phone rings . . .

Diagnosis

His call comes at work; I punch hold and slam the door shut.
"I have bad news. It's cancer."
One hand that looks vaguely like mine holds the
phone to my ear. Another takes notes on
yellow lined paper. Cancer. I write this
word with care, put it in a box; such a
big idea (little Miss Straight A student)
I underline it twice; flash on my need
for a yellow highlighter pen; hear a
voice I think I know beg instead: Give me
something; get me through this day. "Treatable,"
he says. I press the word into my chest.
"what you've got is treatable," sweet lifeline,
I hold on tight: I twist, I spin, I swing.

I hang up the phone. I open the door to my office and walk out into the computer lab, dry eyed and shocky and run a workshop for a group of elementary teachers. I don't know what I taught. I have no idea what they learned. I watch myself do a fairly decent imitation of a sane human being. I spectate on the scene. It's so surreal. I watch all of us at a safe distance, from the far corner of the room.

TREATMENT

The cycle of surgeries begins. A lumpectomy followed by a mastectomy followed by two attempts at reconstruction (one failure, one moderately successful). Scheduled in between the surgeries and short recovery periods, are eight rounds of chemotherapy and six and one-half weeks of radiation. At a very low point trying to cope with the side effects and still keep working, I reach out to a therapist for help:

The therapist listens. Listens to all of it. Listens and nods in places. Murmurs the occasional, "Uh-huh," to keep me talking. With her encouragement, I slowly spill details from my cancer story . . .

I feel the therapist's gaze as I ramble on. Feel her kind gray eyes reading me. Then I sense her focus slowly drift away from my face, up, above my forehead, to stop at an invisible point right above my head. Self-consciously I reach for a handful of hair trailing down the nape of my neck to jerk the wig back into place.

Damn this wig. This long, dark-brown synthetic wig named Jennifer. Named no doubt to distinguish her from wigs called Candy (curly brunette), Jasmine (blonde and straight) or Danielle (wavy red). But with wigs having names, I can sit here in therapy as a newbie cancer survivor and actually whine, "I hate Jennifer. She's itchy and uncomfortable. Plus, she makes me look like a female impersonator, don't you think?" Somehow, in this small room, tastefully decorated in rich, dark wood paneling and flowery chintz slipcovers, I can openly share my worst here-and-now fear with a trained professional: my nightmare that one day at work, Jennifer will take a nose dive right off my head, leaving me standing speechless and humiliated, (not to mention totally bald), in front of an audience full of strangers.

Bottom line, I am trying therapy on for size. To see how it fits. There's no question I need some help. Cancer treatment is wreaking predictable havoc—from the inside out, from the outside in—on my body, my spirit, my life. What's most upsetting is that when I look in the mirror I can't find any "me" that even looks vaguely familiar.

Springsteen's sad song lyrics are starting to make frightening sense: "I was unrecognizable to myself." Maybe cancer has actually changed me into some stranger named Jennifer. Maybe therapy will help me understand this new, disturbing sense of self. Maybe I am trying to put up a good front, playing the part of Super Cancer Patient, but in reality I am slowly losing it. Maybe, just maybe, arm wrestling with appearance demons is a smokescreen for the real life-and-death issues I am unwilling (or unable) to think about right now. Maybe I don't have a clue.

When our first fifty-minute hour comes to an end, the therapist rises from her chair with tears welling up in her eyes and walks the few steps across the room from her chair to mine with her arms opened wide. She draws me into an embrace and hugs me uncomfortably close. Releasing me with a warm pat on the back, she says somberly, "It's not just your cancer. You are part of the community of women who live on this planet. We suffer as you suffer. Fight hard. Fight well. We fight side by side with you."

She sends me out the door with a clear and compelling mission: to go off and fight the Cancer Wars for the Good of Womankind. And maybe because that's such a tall order, such a major agenda item on anyone's "to-do" list, I never make another appointment to see her again. Either that, or I don't need to. After all, I have been given my marching orders for this particularly challenging mission: I am Warrior Woman, and cancer is the enemy I have to beat to a pulp. Looking back, almost six years after the fact, I know that the "cancer script" the therapist handed over that day in her office played itself out, one scene after another, all the way through treatment.

Truth be told, I put so much energy into playing a role, "courageously fighting the good fight," that Sandy, my favorite oncology nurse, made a comment during one of my last chemo infusions that I will never forget. "Ease up on yourself a little bit, why don't you?" she said. "You know, when this is all over, no medals will be given out."

She was so right. When my treatment finally ended, in fact, there were no awards for bravery; there wasn't a medal or ribbon or shiny gold star in sight. But maybe it's just as well. You see, because after cancer treatment —the toxic drugs, the repeat surgeries, the radiation—I didn't have much of a chest left to pin them onto anyway.

WRITING TO HEAL, HEALING TO WRITE

In the two years' time it took me to get through cancer treatment, my journal grew to over 100 pages. I documented my time in CancerLand, from diagnosis to recovery with anecdotes, bad jokes, lists, rambling streams of consciousness, and letters that I would never ever send. The form varied and most times didn't matter much at all. I wrote. I rewrote. I cried, blew my nose, cried again, dried my eyes, then wrote some more. Sometimes using "I"; other times a royal "we." The most satisfying writing was done using third person. As "she" I could be miles away from what was happening to "me." Whatever emotion bubbled up—fear, anger, grief for the many losses, shame —whatever was burning inside of me found its way out and onto the page. I lived alone and chose to keep my diagnosis a secret from all but my small inner circle of family and closest "bosom buddies." So, my laptop computer immediately became my new best friend, always alert, empathetic and on stand-by, sitting patiently at the dining room table, eagerly awaiting my next daily update.

I ultimately printed out the journal and sorted the writing into sections with illustrative chapter headings: *Slash* for my six surgeries. *Poison* described eight rounds of chemotherapy. *Burn* documented my radiation treatments. I three-hole punched the pages and filed them away in a binder, at one point believing that the journal had served its healing purpose. But that wasn't to be the case at all.

Over the years my CancerLand journal has been the well that I have returned to again and again for the raw materials resulting in the more polished pieces that I later published online. At the time that I was creating the journal, I truly thought it was an end in itself. But the real healing gradually emerged from revisiting those initial impressions, reshaping them and ultimately sharing them with different audiences.

I have always been a lover of reading and writing. As an adolescent I kept a diary. (But what teenage girl didn't?) During adolescence I was drawn to the romance of poetry and remember writing a poem for my first high school boyfriend. I can even recall as a teenager imitating Edna St. Vincent Millay once or twice. In college, I was one of those English majors who wondered how I could possibly earn a living with only a passion for reading and writing as my potentially marketable skill set. At least I had the basic tools of literacy in place when I truly needed them, after a cancer diagnosis.

Looking back, though, I can clearly see that my journal entries were shaped by the cancer memoirs, the so-called "sick lit" that I began to collect and read somewhat obsessively once I got tired of all the medical literature I absorbed after diagnosis. Two of my favorite memoirs were Joyce Wadler's *My Breast* and Katherine Russell Rich's *The Red Devil*. Here were single women who told stories of survivorship that I could relate to.

THE PINK RIBBON POETS

Ultimately it was the breast cancer poetry that resonated most loudly for me. Alicia Ostriker's *Mastectomy Poems* were a revelation. I stumbled upon an excerpt online and immediately had to buy her book, *The Crack in Everything*, where all the mastectomy poems were included. What an epiphany: other women had taken this journey, somehow gotten through it with their souls and spirit intact and then, almost miraculously, had turned their trauma into high art. The ultimate lemons-into-lemonade strategy. If I couldn't become an instant card-carrying member of this exclusive club, I could at least try on the role for size and see what it felt like. My shelves slowly filled with the cancer poetry of Hilda Raz, Audre Lorde, Anne Silver, Helene Davis, and Lois Hjelmstad. I read *Art.Rage.Us* cover to cover. I stalked Amazon.com and used Google to hunt down more of these so-called pink ribbon poets. Survivor poetry deeply touched and inspired me. It's no surprise that my first efforts involved imitating those poets whose work I most admired.

It's hard to remember precisely when I started experimenting with my journal entries, turning them into poems masquerading as "almost sonnets" (fourteen lines long, ten beats to a line). I called them "ten by fourteens" and the syllable counting of the form I had created quieted my mind and gave me some relief.

If there was a demon to wrestle, it wasn't the cancer itself. One of my worst demons was making peace with my physical self, my "new normal" after treatment ended. So much had changed. What I looked like. How uncomfortable I felt in my own skin, walking around in a body that had been so dramatically altered. Then there was the day I realized that dressing this new body of mine had become a daily form of torture, an ongoing painful reminder of all the losses that were piling up (*nothing fits, nothing feels right, nothing looks right*). I stared longingly at my favorite blue sweater dress hanging in the closet, knowing that I would never be able to wear it again and sat down at the computer to write about that feeling in my journal. This "ten by

70

fourteen" poem grew from that entry some time later:

Symmetry in the Blue Dress

The blue dress hangs in the closet on a
padded hanger, under plastic to keep
the shoulders round. It's a sweater dress with
buttons down the front, a deep vee neck style.
Such a wonderful dress, deep navy blue,
designed to wrap the body in a warm
wool hug. Rich. Elegant. Timeless. Classic.
The blue dress hangs in the closet and mocks
me as a relic of who I was and
what my body used to look like. Before.
Such a simple dream actually. Me
in the blue dress standing in front of the
mirror, fooling the onlooker with my
cosmetic sleight of hand, both sides matching.

Before long, I began experimenting with concrete poems as well, letting the shape of the words on the page resonate along with the content.[4] Once again, it was a journal entry that inspired me.

Many cancer survivors vividly remember and write about the traumatic moment when the bandages are removed following a mastectomy. Some immediately stare at the scar where their breast used to be and bravely begin to move towards acceptance. Others wrestle with denial, turning away, refusing to look at their disfigurement.

With multiple reconstructive surgeries over the years, a different plastic surgeon each time, I have struggled with agonizing repeat "unveilings" of my upper body. And each time when a procedure is done and the bandages are removed days afterwards, I have critically judged the result and asked myself a question that still has no clear answer: *Can I ever make peace with how breast cancer has forever altered me?* After one of my most difficult and extensive surgical revisions, I received some "practical advice" from a family member that upset me so much I immediately jotted it down in my journal and much later turned

71

it into a very satisfying poem in the shape of a woman:

Survivor's Guide to Post-Operative Body Image

if the

scars

upset

you

that

much

she said,

just stop

looking

at them.

you can

take a

shower

without

looking

down.

yes

you

can.

When treatment finally ends there's the challenge of getting on with life. It's not getting back to normal. That's not possible. Too much has happened. Too much has changed. For cancer survivors, it's more like getting used to a "new normal." Writing continues to help me cope with the demon of what can't be controlled. A prose poem describing the twice a year visit to the oncologist captures what that experience feels like:

Six Month Check-up

My six month check-up is almost over. And so far it's been business as usual.

I've been weighed and measured. We've been through the "are-there-any-lumps-bumps-or-bruises" routine. (Classic cancer exam questions. Asked and answered. Check). The doctor has also finished his dance of the fingertips across the lymph nodes on my neck. A six-month check-up means getting stuck for blood, means warm hands pressing down, means poking around, means an all-out search up and down, for signs of "the enemy" above or below the waist. My six-month check-up is almost over. Now maybe my heart can stop its panicky racing and slow down and sound somewhat closer to normal. Not that there's anything normal about being treated by an oncologist. I'm nervous for days beforehand. I'm jumpy once I step off the elevator on the fourth floor of the hospital. So right about now I'm ready to exhale already. I want to get dressed. I want to be somewhere else. (anywhere else, to tell you the truth). My six-month check-up is almost over. The oncologist washes his hands at the sink, his back to me as I sit on the examining table holding the edges of the salmon-colored gown together over my bare chest. I hear the doctor's voice over the splashing sounds of the water as he soaps up, "Everything looks good," he says, reaching for a paper towel. "In fact, your blood counts are high enough for you to get chemo today." And with one simple sentence I am a survivor sucked back in time from this reality into another, from here and now back to there and then, to this same room, this same scene five years prior when a baby blue barcalounger in the Chemo Lounge down the hall was in fact the next stop after the check-up and a crude noise sounding a bit like "no" chokes its way up out of my throat where it hangs in the air between us. The oncologist smiles at the joke he's just played on me.

Another poem I wrote helps me deal with the anniversary of my diagnosis. Every fall, I pay a return visit to the radiologist who first located my tumor for a repeat mammogram of my remaining breast. As the day approaches, I joke about returning to "the scene of the crime." But it's little more than bravado.

One Good Thing About My Yearly Mammogram

I'm in
and out of
there, I swear,
in the blink of an
eye. Moving at warp
speed, clothes peeled to
the waist in seconds flat.
Motion lines blur, tremble
on either side of me. I fight
off demons that recur, mute
their evil chatter (we found it
once, we'll find it again). Steal
a quick glance down at my
watch. It's official: I'm in
and out and on my way,
I'd say in maybe half
the time it takes
everybody else.

My yearly mammogram brings me face to face with the frightening specter of recurrence. Poetry continues to help me cope as that anniversary comes around again on the calendar. I confess that the flattened breast shape of the poem pleases me immensely; I have finally stopped apologizing for my newly morbid sense of humor. It's just another side effect of where my travels in CancerLand have taken me.

"Writing about Boris and plotting his imminent demise helped me wrestle with my first real demon—that I had no control. . . . Never had, never would. Over anything related to cancer, which by its very definition, means life out of control." Alysa writes first and foremost to exercise control and freedom. She plays with form and structure in con-

crete poems and villanelles and when she wields a pen, she has a sense of mastery and total control. She navigates skillfully in the safety of journal territory, in which she alone is the master cartographer. Her pen serves as compass and the lines of her journal signify the distance she has traveled.

The journey to CancerLand is harrowing, filled with terror and uncertainty. It is like walking in the dark through a tunnel. Yet in this tunnel, Alysa hears the voices of other strong women who have traveled this passage before her. She reads and writes in kinship with her literary friends—Audre Lorde, Alicia Ostriker, and many others— reassured that she is not alone on this journey.[5] She gleans courage from their stories and poetry. Alysa reads and writes for the purpose of self-nurturance, inspired by the bravery, humor and ability of women writers to remain passionate despite cancer.

The act of taking time every day actually becomes a ritual to "digest" the events that have occurred, no matter how unpalatable and unpleasant. Although many doctors in CancerLand ask the question, "How do you feel?" they are asking about the physical realm. Through the ritual of daily writing, Alysa has the opportunity to give expression to the emotional dimension of her life. Writing simultaneously expresses and contains her intense emotions, achieving the important purpose of self-regulation.

Through the shifting of time, space, and matter, Alysa chooses to return to particular focal points that are then subjected to her humor, her sharp sensitivity, and sometimes her scorn. During the cancer journey, with its endless rounds of exams, lab tests, and drug protocols, it is not uncommon for the patient to feel that she is a specimen or object. With her writing process, Alysa effectively turns the tables. In an act of mastery, the doctors, the therapist, and even relatives all are studied and often quite harshly judged under her probing gaze.

Alysa captures her traumatic journey by externalizing and concretizing thoughts and feelings on paper. This externalization makes her experience available for reflection, witnessing, and integration. The process of writing helps her to integrate dissonant aspects of her journey. As the cells of her body are dying and regenerating, another trans-formation is taking place. Alysa's creativity is an assertive action to counteract the process of destruction that has taken place in her body. Cancerland is a place that not even the most adventurous of travelers would want to visit. However, Alysa's greetings from Cancerland carry news of the ultimate outcome: healing, recovery, and renewal.

~ 4 ~

The Journal That Was an Anchor
Joel Gabriel

There is a saying "Sticks and stones may break my bones, but names can never harm me." Unfortunately, it's not true. While over a million children are physically abused each year, millions more are verbally abused. Words may leave scars and wounds that are felt for a lifetime.[1]

Children who grow up in hostile environments are subjected to conditions that seriously affect the way they see themselves, others, and the world. Psychologists are quick to point out that we learn what we see, and parents' behavior makes up our first templates, the blueprints for our earliest thoughts and feelings. What if our parents are less than perfect—and they always are! What if a role model is consistently under great stress and exhibits disturbed and unhealthy behavior?

This is the story of one very resilient and persevering child and how he found ways—through the written and spoken word—to transform himself, despite a difficult childhood, into the kind of person he wanted to be. This is Joel's story.

77

THE EARLY YEARS—BROKEN TRUST

I n folklore there is a tale about a storyteller with a large bag on his back filled with story after story. The story that I need to tell you is a story lying at the bottom of the bag. It is a dark and musty story, and my least favorite. However, I have learned that sharing this story is healing. The story is an affirmation of my pain and must come out of hiding. It is scary for me to share this, but it brings the shadows of my life out into the light and disempowers my demons.

It is Chicago, 1970. The neighborhood is Bridgeport, a working-class area of Chicago. A five-year-old Mexican-American boy is playing Spiderman on a chain link fence with his sister. They hear mom calling them to come in to dinner but they're having too much fun to pay attention. After the third yell, they reluctantly walk into the kitchen of the basement apartment. Mom is standing frozen in place with a look of fury in her eyes. She stands like Medusa, fury slowly turning into rage, as the children's confusion turns into terror. The kitchen table stands between her and the frightened and confused children. "Que hicimos? (What did we do?) Por que estas tan enojada? (Why are you so angry?)"

A knife suddenly appears in her hand. She chants a mantra, through clenched furious teeth. "Los voy a matar! Los voy a matar!" (I am going to kill you!)

The children start to scream, their eyes fixed on the large kitchen knife. But they do not move. The boy is transfixed by the face of Medusa that has suddenly replaced the face of his mother. Her hair has changed into snakes. Her eyes are blood red in rage. She points the knife at the children, who start to scream in terror. The children's screams bring the father running in. "Que pasa?! Que haces?!" He sees the knife and runs over to the mother, grabbing her wrist.

"Ya! Ya! Esta bien! Esta bien!" (Okay! Okay! Everything is okay!) He calms her down. The snakes disappear. Her eyes change back. She realizes what she has done, and begins to sob. She embraces her children and asks for forgiveness. The little boy half embraces and half hates her. From that moment on, trust is broken. Something is forever altered.

Never again would there be a feeling of safety after that . . . not for a very long time. Mom suffered from severe clinical depression that in its most extreme form manifested in dissociative psychotic rage. I often found myself living in the unpredictable world of my mother's moods. Sometimes she was calm and at peace, usually when she was cooking for the family, but at other times she would lash out venomously at perceived offenses, slights, or challenges. We became her caretakers. I learned to walk on eggshells, learned how to intuit her every mood. I became hyperaware of mood shifts, ready to anticipate any earthquakes or sudden movements. Pops wasn't around much of the time. He sometimes worked seven days a week, fourteen hours a day as a janitor in a meatpacking plant. His love for us was boundless, but he could not protect us.

Although she was always present physically, she would frequently stare into space with a vacant look in her eyes, and I knew that she was not really there. At other times, she was ridiculing and belittling. When I would bring her an idea, an exciting possibility, she would dismiss it as silly, stupid, or ridiculous. In anticipation of her throwing my thoughts in the garbage, I started to have difficulty speaking. My words got stuck; they were tired of hitting a wall of frustration and anger. As a way to stop communicating with her, I developed a severe stutter, which further infuriated her, and made the stutter worse. In school, I received straight A's. I was loved by my teachers and held up as a model student.

I started to consciously make myself into the good boy so as not to be hurt. I became a people pleaser. Don't make waves. Don't upset anyone. Don't get anyone angry. Swallow your own angry feelings. This was my way to survive. I pushed down my feelings with food, and became a fat little boy. However, a part of me thrived.

My inner life was rich and imaginative. I had a thirst for knowledge and a burning curiosity about everything. I began acting in high school theater and found it was the perfect venue to express emotion and receive applause and validation. No stutter there. I continued my acting, receiving a B.A. in theater from University of Illinois at Chicago. I trained at the London Academy of Music and Dramatic Arts in London on a Fulbright Scholarship, and eventually received my MFA in Acting from Columbia University. I loved being in the spotlight even though at heart I was still a shy person. Theater gave me a way to temporarily vanquish my insecurities and receive validation.

In my late twenties, I discovered that writing in a journal gave me a sense of control. It seemed to help me to regulate my own emotions. I started writing on a daily basis. The journal provided me with a totally safe place to sort through the events of the day at my own pace. It gave me a third eye with which to examine the world. With this third eye, I felt empowered and better able to understand myself and others. Like a non-judgmental mother, the journal could hold all my thoughts and feelings for me; that was something my mother had not been able to do. The journal held my dreams, nightmares, thoughts, poems, and unsent letters.

One of my therapists called it a love object. Indeed, my journal was always there for me. It anchored my feelings and grounded me. For a period of about fifteen years, I did not miss a day of journaling. My writing chronicles my awkward struggles to overcome my insecurities. It bears witness in black and white to the invisible power of terror and its remnants of betrayal and confusion.

THE TIES THAT BIND

I've always known what I wanted and have always followed my heart, trying to grow into the person I was meant to be. In this I have been fearless. But do you remember the first dark story that I told you? It still cast a shadow across my life. In therapy and in my writing, I was to revisit this story again and again. It's thirty-five years later, and I still think about the knife in Medusa's hand.

Journal Entry—May 26, 2000
Dear Mom,
How could you do this? Why did you do this? I am still trying to forgive you for the pain you caused me. Your instability throughout my childhood permanently imprinted me with a sense of impending doom, terror, and fear. I was a child—and so

were you. If things didn't go your way, you would throw your tantrum, you would make your displeasure known by degrading us, insulting us, or just manipulating us in some way, whether through guilt or anger. How many times a day in my early teen years did you repeat over and over how fat I was, with a look of disgust on your face? I hated you for your intolerance and lack of understanding. I don't know if you knew that I ate even more just to spite you, to have some way to get back at you for your resentment. Even though the adult Joel wants to forgive, the wounded Joel still cries out. . . . Whenever you gave affection, it always came at a price. I would sometimes cringe at your touch, because it was needy, or was attached to some form of manipulation or guilt. How could I trust you? On the other hand, even as a very small boy, I saw you suffering and felt very helpless. I both resented and was angry at you and also felt deep sadness for you when you were depressed. . . . I was always losing you to depression, to those blanked out stares that were so common as I was growing up.

Even when you were present, you often did not really see me.

Do you even know who I am? . . .

Fear of abandonment was entwined with my fear of intimacy. The knife cut into the trust that should be part of a normal, loving relationship. For many years, I suffered from hypervigilance in relationships, and was subject to feelings of intense jealousy based on a neediness that cried for total attentiveness and validation. Sleep issues of restlessness and disturbing dreams of violence and aggression haunted me. I later learned that these are symptoms of PTSD—Post Traumatic Stress Disorder.

Journal Entry—June 12, 1998
The Fox and the Bull Dream

I was on the outside of an enclosed fence area. There was a fox on the outside with me. The fox was harassing a bull on the inside area of the fence. The bull was trying to get the fox. It was very angry. The fox would run around the outside of the fence with the bull in pursuit. The scene changed to the fox being inside the fence area with the bull. I was still on the outside.

The fox was harassing the bull even more cruelly now, the bull was getting angrier and angrier. At the end of the dream, the bull was chasing the fox at full speed. Just as the bull reached the fox, the fox pulled out a knife and slashed at the bull underneath its legs. The bull let out an unearthly bellow that was a combination of all the frustration it had felt up to that point at not catching the fox, and the pain it felt as the knife slashed through its groin. I felt so much empathy for the bull that I woke up sobbing.

It is clear to me that this is a dream about masculinity and castration. It is a dream that is burned into my psyche. The appearance of the knife mirrors the original incident. I was fearless in taking on challenges in other aspects of my life. I succeeded in attaining my professional goals. I have loving relationships with good friends, and a beautiful apartment overlooking the Hudson River in New York. But in this one area—in the search for my life partner—I continue to be stymied, often returning again and again to my relationship with my mother. Even if a relationship began well, issues of trust would eventually surface. I feared abandonment; secretly I wondered when a knife would appear in my girlfriend's hands, the knife as a symbol for a sudden betrayal, a horrible desertion.

FINDING MY VOICE

I began to go to therapy, instinctively choosing a female therapist to work on forming a trusting relationship with a woman. I continued my journal writing as a self-help tool. At times, I brought my writing to my therapist, and we would explore it further. My therapy had a strong narrative element in it, and in-between sessions, there was sometimes a flurry of e-mail writing that enabled me to continue an ongoing dialogue with a female who was consistent, attentive, and unconditionally caring. In addition to talk therapy, art, role-play, and poetry, I sometimes taped parts of a session and transcribed it later. Writing things down seemed to give credence to my thoughts and feelings.

In therapy, I often referred to feelings of constriction, of ties binding me to my family of origin. During one session, to my amazement, my therapist took out a spool of black thread, and with my permission, she proceeded to wrap me, many times over with this thread.

Journal Entry—Nov. 16, 2001

> *Therapist: How do you feel?*
>
> *Joel: I feel very close to the, uh . . . I feel sad . . . sad.*
>
> *Therapist: What's making you sad?*
>
> *Joel: The fact that I'm still tied up like this.*
>
> *Therapist: Well, you don't have to be tied up like this. I'd like you to look at each strand, and tell me what it might represent. The ties that bind you to your mother . . . the negative ties that bind you. Then you're going to use your hands to cut each strand after you name it, okay?*
>
> *Joel: This seems to be . . . these three . . . around my neck . . . connected to my throat . . . the pain of not being able to do anything for her.*
>
> *Therapist: Helplessness? Okay, are you willing to let go of the pain of not being able to save her?*
>
> *Joel: I'm READY to let go. Yes.*
>
> *Therapist: Are you sure?*
>
> *Joel: Yes.*
>
> *Therapist: I want you to cut the string. You'll also let go of the helpless feeling because you're choosing to keep that helplessness right now.*
>
> *Joel: So, this is the way that I'm still plugged in to that?*
>
> *Therapist: Right. And all of these three are connected to that. Could you define or name each one specifically? I am bound to her . . .*
>
> *Joel: With this one I am bound to her . . . uh . . . through tears.*
>
> *Therapist: I choose to cut . . . I choose to cut . . .*
>
> *Joel: The string that's binding me to her through tears . . . (sound of scissors cutting string).*
>
> *Therapist: And the second string?*
>
> *Joel: This is . . . the string that's binding me to her . . . this is the need to please her . . .*
>
> *Therapist: Okay. Are you willing to relinquish your need to please?*
>
> *Joel: Yes. I am willing to relinquish the need to please. (snip)*

Therapist: And this one under your armpit?

Joel: This one under my armpit is . . . the need to be comforted by her.

Therapist: Near your heart.

Joel: It's like a hug.

Therapist: Go ahead. Are you ready to relinquish the need to be comforted by her?

Joel: Yes, I relinquish this string, which is the need to be comforted by her. (snip)

Therapist: You still have something around your neck. What is that?

Joel: This is the suppressed anger.

Therapist: Mm hmm. And do you push down?

Joel: The anger I push down . . . the anger that I swallow when I have to deal with her.

Therapist: What will you do with the anger instead of swallowing it?

Joel: Uhhh . . . I want to say transform it in some way . . .

Therapist: Instead of swallowing it, and having it go down, you could . . .

Joel: I could have it come up . . . express it in a healthy way.

Therapist: Okay. (snip)

After the session, I felt like a puppet whose strings had been cut. Maybe like a newborn. But, of course, cutting loose from the ties of emotional bondage was, in reality, not so simple. My conflicts would play themselves out on the stage of real life. I came to see reflections of my mother in every female with whom I became intimate.

Sharon was my first girlfriend. We were in our early twenties. She was a very angry, cynical young woman who lived in a dark house. Her father had abandoned the family years before. Sharon sulked, pouted, pointed out flaws, and was hypercritical, like Mom. She was self-absorbed and bitterly enmeshed in her own troubled family situation. Eventually, I realized that I didn't want this negative energy. I didn't want the disparaging remarks and the feeling of angry entitlement. I felt that it was killing a part of me—the part of me that had always been there, the part that genuinely loved people and took joy in life.

Sharon was a younger version of Mom, the little girl who wanted to be taken care of. Perhaps that's what I bought into. It made me feel like Pops, taking care of the weak little woman. Sharon literally became a little girl at times, and wanted to be seen as someone adorable who needed protection. So, I played Daddy, and she was Mommy. We played these roles for four years, until I understood that the connection was damaging my ability to love life itself. Anger was our commonality. Anger and the yearning for love despite our wounds. We fed off of each other's rages.

Journal Entry—February 10, 1987

The Glowing Coal

A piece of coal
rests deep inside my soul.
handed down,
from man to man, to ME.
It glows deep red.
I drizzle it with water.
I feel the sizzle and the fizzle.
smoke catches in my throat, makes my eyes
water . . .

> *water*
What kind of water will work
to keep the bright, red glowing coal
under control?

Here was someone as angry as I was! I was able to break free. To not do so would have crippled me emotionally.

After a welcomed period of solitude, I became involved with Patricia, who was beautiful but depressed. Her face often wore a remote, wooden mask of sadness. Patricia suffered from moods of depression like Mom. Her face would dissolve into a cloud. The eyes would become vacant. I wanted to shake her sometimes and say, "Where are you? You've gone away again." I would feel rageful after her absences. I lived with Patricia for a year and a half.

I wanted to rescue her from her dismal journeys, where her body was present but her soul was elsewhere. One summer night we had a terrible fight and I stormed out of the apartment. When I returned, I found her in the bathtub, having drunk vodka and slashed her wrists with a razor blade. When I think of Patricia, I think of her disappearing into the fog, her face dissolving into a cloud. I could not save her.

Journal Entry—March 30, 1991

Grief, My Friend
I feel sad but grief
is my friend who
has been with me since I was
small
Grief, I like your safe,
enveloping arms—
You were my first blanket.

Patricia reflected my mother's sadness and her deep, destructive anger. We understood each other's grief, but grief was the cement in the relationship, and it was toxic. I finally broke away.

I was, once again, relieved to live a solitary life (solitary was safe!), but not for long. Eventually, I was seduced by Yvette, an uninhibited artist, a Bohemian woman who was unlike any of the women I had ever known. In sharp contrast to my own conservative parents, Yvette was the daughter of two European hippies from the Woodstock era. A relationship with Yvette was a rebellion against everything familiar. However, I was not in control of my emotions. Yvette was very sexually uninhibited. I found myself becoming highly jealous of the attention she gave to an old boyfriend, and the time she spent on her art projects. I became the stereotype of the jealous Latin lover, possessive and accusing. Now that I think of it, this was very similar to some of the screaming matches I heard between my mother and father as I was growing up. My father, like many Latino men, was possessive, and there was often a feeling of suspicion and accusations of infidelity in the house.

Journal Entry—June 1, 1999

> *The green fire wells up in my chest,*
> *A blast furnace of anger and anxiety.*
> *She walks hand in hand with an old flame,*
> *Now a friend.*
> *But how,*
> *Can a once-lover's flashing fire,*
> *Turn to harmless ashes?*
> *Escalating Jealousy! 4-alarm madness!*

It seemed to me that every man Yvette would greet on the street as a friend was a threat to me as a man. Her best friend, Paul, was a man she had known since undergraduate school, and I felt that they had an uncomfortably close physical relationship, hugging and kissing, at times holding hands as we walked down the street. Yvette assured me that it was innocent, but somehow my jealousy and possessiveness became worse. One day, Yvette confessed to me that, before we had met, she and Paul had slept together as an experiment to find out if they were compatible as lovers. From that moment on, the jealousy took on a life of its own, creating scenarios in my mind, and torturing me with visions of Yvette sleeping with strangers. The green monster finally destroyed the relationship, and Yvette broke up with me. After Yvette, I swore myself to celibacy, which lasted for about one year.

Finally, I met Roberta. She was open, loving, creative, and very intelligent. She did not appear to be in any way dysfunctional. We fell in love and planned a future together. But after a year of living together, we found that we were not so compatible. I think my unhealthy desire to please her caused me to bend excessively, but I still couldn't bend backwards as far as she wanted without breaking. Compromise was difficult. If she wanted to go out, I wanted to stay in. If I wanted to paint the room blue, she wanted green. Once again, I found myself trying to please and placate. Roberta would take out her frustrations on me and our interactions would escalate into drama. I hated that dynamic. It was the dynamic that existed in my childhood home. I kept trying to make the relationship work.

For a while, we were getting by. And then one day, Roberta was very anxious about a project she was working on. I remember us sitting on the floor talking. She held a teacup, speaking about her frustration. Her tension and insecurity escalated, and she slammed the teacup onto the floor, yelling. She worked herself into a rage, and I felt helpless. I watched her face—the face of Medusa, the same look on my mother's face when she held the knife.

All of the women I dated wore my mom's face in one way or another. However, I had the feeling that it was all too easy blaming Mom. I needed to explore the role my father had played, and I started to examine the Latino role model that was my legacy.

I wrote an unsent letter to my father that was five pages long. Here is an excerpt:

Journal Entry—February 20, 2003

Dear Pops,

In many ways, the pain I feel at the dynamic we have is greater than the pain I feel with Mom. With Mom, I feel a deep anger and rage. With you, I feel the pain of absence.

Everything about you is hidden to me. I only know a small part of you. From what I know, and the stories you tell me about your eighty-three years on this earth, you have gone through the life experiences of five men. But despite the incredible amount of living that you have been through, you are closed off, and a large part of you has become resentful, bitter, cynical, and mean. Why do I feel that I am, in some ways, a less than ideal son to you? Perhaps this is illogical, because you recently told me how proud you are of my accomplishments. Why do I feel unworthy in your eyes? Maybe because we never became friends. In some very basic way, we don't trust one another.

I know your father died an alcoholic at a young age and I have heard stories of you dragging your father out of the gutter in Mexico. I know that you lost your first wife. But do I have siblings that I am unaware of? Why are you so secretive? I think this is why we never became friends. You never let me in. But you did your duty, what is required of every Mexican man: you provided for us. But where are you? Who are you?

I also have a strong gut feeling that you were quite a ladies' man and a womanizer. Every Mexican man is expected to be. But I resent you for the way you treated Mom. The whole Mexican power machismo trip is poison. It is a legacy I have inherited. You have imprinted me with your rage and impatience.

I remember you saying that your grandfather's family lost everything in the Mexican Revolution because my grandfather was "on the wrong side." I have a very clear image of the story you told me about when you were about five years old. The family was in hiding because of the war, and your father had to remain in hiding. My grandma took you to the roof of a building where your father was standing on the roof of an adjoining building. She told you, "That's your father. Wave to him." He waved at you, and you waved back. This story is very sad. Your father was hidden to you, just as you are hidden to me . . .

WEAVING MY OWN IDENTITY

I was very different from my immediate family, the only one to have an education beyond high school. I thrived on Shakespeare and the classics. I wanted to be a person of the world, and I sought every opportunity to learn. I was drawn to other people like myself, who loved reading and culture, music, theater, and ideas. The larger world called to me, and I responded.

I came from a marginalized culture, and as first-generation, my sense of self was fragmented. Who was I? Mexican? American? Both? Mixed? What do I keep? What do I discard? I had to reweave my identity. In my thirties I began a deep spiritual search. I studied Eastern spirituality, including Taoism and Buddhism. However, upon arriving in New York to attend graduate school, I found that Judaism called deeply to my soul. After researching my family and questioning my father, he revealed that his side of the family had been Anousim, Crypto-Jews (Marranos) who had been forced to convert to Catholicism after the Spanish expulsion of 1492. It all made sense. So, after studying for a few years, I converted to Judaism. I asked for and received my family's generous acceptance of who I had become. Additionally, my father seemed to reconnect to this part of himself after my conversion.

One day I was on the subway in New York, when a troubled teen came over to me and started to talk. He asked me if he could go home with me because he had no place to go. My heart went out to him. Subsequently, I volunteered to become a Big Brother. Later I worked in Project Liberty after 9/11. Working with people in distress touched me deeply. I found a part of myself capable of deep empathy and connection. From being an actor (speaking words) to being a speech teacher (helping others find their voice), I came to a profession of listening—that of the therapist. In 2006, I acquired a Masters in Clinical Social Work.

MENDING

At some point, I recognized that I needed to look beyond the stereotypes of the absent father, the hysterical mother, and Joel, the victim. I needed to make an honest effort to know my parents and to see the whole picture. I went home one Christmas, and found myself in my mother's guest room. I found the atmosphere suffocating. But to my surprise, I noted the beautiful green plants in the room. A week later, I told my therapist, "These plants know something about my mother that I don't know."

My therapist said, "Great first line of a poem. Let's both do one now, with that as the first line." And we both wrote.

Journal Entry—January 5th, 2004

The Plant Poem by Joel
These plants know something about my mom
Something I don't know.

They get her in ways I don't.
Maybe they don't mind her attention—how do they accept her love
  without wilting?
On the contrary,
They are vibrant, healthy, green, shiny. They take the milk of
  human kindness.
Why couldn't I?
The proof of her pure energy and love
  lives in them.

My therapist wrote the following:

> *These plants know something*
>   *about my Mom*
> *Something I don't know*
> *Something I forgot . . .*
>
> *Was I a plant that could*
>   *not do*
> *Whatever it is that you*
>   *wanted me to?*
> *Did you not notice me*
>   *wanting care?*
> *I begged for a presence*
> *That was not there.*
>
> *The plants are healthy*
>   *green and bright*
> *Somewhere in your soul*
>   *They find a light*
> *That shines and brings to life*
>   *This Green*
> *The lushest plants*
>   *I've ever seen*

The plants know something
about my Mom
Something I forgot
They know her tender touch
That soothes
While she patiently coaxes
Never disapproves

I saw my own poem as sad. It filled me with grief and longing. Certainly, the fear and disapproval in my childhood environment had not been conducive to my growth. I was almost envious of the plants and the love they received from Mom. I felt, in comparison, unloved. On the other hand, in my therapist's poem, there was no question that the mother loved the child. This thought surprised me. It raised a question in me. "How can I take in the healthy part of her love and *not* take in that which is toxic?"

Before this, I experienced my mother as completely toxic, and, therefore, I had rejected her for survival reasons. The plants and their healthy survival, however, became the symbol for something healthy that could possibly exist in her presence. It helped me to consider new ways of thinking about and interacting with my mother and father.

Journal Entry—April 15, 2005

Dear Mom and Dad,
I am beginning to see that you are making a real effort to change as you grow older. I sense more love and acceptance from you lately, even if you don't understand me or my life completely. You are growing too. I think I need to let my defenses down in order to accept you now.
Mom, I understand that you were suffering. Pops was never around. You had to carry the burden all by yourself. Of course it was hard. In the ideal world, I could say, "Why weren't you stronger? Why weren't you as strong as some of the beautifully strong women I know in my life now?" But you weren't. And that's not your fault.

Communication has been impossible. (It is still inconceivable to me that you yelled at me for stuttering!) But I will keep trying. With this in mind, I am going to try a new experiment with you and Pops. . . . I am going to begin to speak more English with you. You may find this strange, but it is a way to reclaim my ground. Unfortunately, Spanish and the Mexican culture has also been tainted for me with the pain of my childhood.

I need to communicate to you through the safety of English, my language. I am different now, very different than the boy you lived with. I have made my choices. But I don't want to shut you out.

Mom, there is a good memory of us together that has stayed with me my whole life. We are outside, in the big yard of the basement apartment on Thirty-Third Street. We are sitting on the steps, you have a blade of grass in your hand and are showing it to me, maybe trying to teach me something about it. We are studying it. I feel your love for me as we sit there. You are gentle, nurturing, calm. I feel very safe. I hope we can begin to love one another the way we were meant to love one another when I was growing up.

Pop, I have an ancient memory of us in Mexico . . . I couldn't have been more than two or three. We are traveling from place to place, You are taking me to the haunts you used to frequent as a young man, insanely happy and proud of me, showing me off to your friends. "This is my son! Look! This is my son!" Your friends are happy for you, They shower me with oohs and ahhs. This feeling you had for me back then hasn't changed. It is still the same pride. I know your love and pride for me is boundless. Without your unconditional love, I couldn't have survived. You are still my rock.

Love,
Joel

TRANSFORMATION

Remember my first terrible story? Did you ever think the boy could become a happy man? And yet, I am happy. That is what I love about stories . . . that if you don't like the one you are in, you can change it. There was so much I didn't like in my original story, that I have created a new one, again and again. I continue to work on my story and my family's story. And I am still searching for my great love. But that's another story.

"As an adult, I found myself so haunted by my parents and my geography that I have spent a lifetime trying to write my way out of my addiction to their memory."[2] *Although these are the words of Pat Conroy, they perfectly describe Joel's predicament. Joel spent many years dealing with his mother's depression, her helplessness, and her ridicule. His father was often absent, working. Home was a hotbed of emotion. Joel's life often felt out of control.*

Joel needed to create a locus of control (mastery), a way to anchor his experience, and subject it to his own scrutiny. Journaling became the natural way to process life events. In the safety of his own home, at a regular time of his choosing, Joel initiated the ritual of writing in order to witness each day and understand its significance. The five freedoms that Virginia Satir wrote about—"the freedom to know what you know, feel what you feel, to say what you feel and think, to ask for what you want, and to take risks on your own behalf"[3]—were all violated for Joel as a child. Writing was an act of restoration of these freedoms.

It is clear in Joel's story that the specter of distrust from childhood invades his romantic relationships. As a child, Joel was flooded by different feelings and often had no one to turn to. The journal is a constant love object, attentive to all of his emotions and thoughts. Through writing and venting without fear of retribution, Joel is creating the most important relationship of trust that there is—he is creating a relationship with himself. He writes for the purpose of self-articulation and identity affirmation. Through the journal, one part of Joel asks a question, another part answers. Because he can see his thoughts in black and white, he can dialogue with himself. By developing and using his observing ego, Joel is able to distance himself, reflect upon his thoughts and feelings, and develop perspective. This process helps Joel to identify and regulate his emotions with greater ease. He is actually learning that he can befriend and trust himself. In theories of social referencing, babies and young children refer back to the parent's faces for approval or disapproval; Joel's mother may not have been a reliable social reference, but the journal is.

Joel started therapy with me at the age of thirty-six. His goal: to have a "normal" intimate and lasting relationship with a woman. His therapy included talk therapy, role-play, and a myriad of creative arts therapy techniques. In addition to intensive weekly sessions, we incorporated narrative therapy. Joel would occasionally ask for a summary or transcript of an important session. These transcripts and summaries helped Joel to fully integrate what had transpired in session. E-mail also gave me the opportunity to highlight pivotal points in the therapy and validate Joel's progress. In addition, Joel could e-mail me at any time and receive a response shortly after. Joel had never experienced this constancy and unconditional acceptance. His trust in me grew. I had the privilege of being the first woman that he was able to trust in his adult life. He was eventually able to transfer this trust to women in general. In fact, Joel is getting married this June.

Time-shifting takes place when Joel returns over and over to the trauma scene of his mother threatening with a knife. Incapable of processing what was happening to him as a child, he experiences flashbacks, a common occurrence for PTSD victims. Writing forces the brain to slow down, and helps trauma victims to process memories that have not been fully integrated. Joel is able to use time-shifting, not only to process the negative memories, but to return to positive memories and to quilt together the fragments of his childhood to make himself whole.

Spoken and written words have always played an important role in Joel's life. As a child he excelled in reading aloud, unimpeded by his stutter. Later, building on this strength, he became an actor, no doubt feeling satisfied when he could mesmerize and capture the attention of *his audience (an impossibility when growing up). Joel was in therapy with me for about five years during which time I saw him transform from a person who was often anxious and sad into a person of greater confidence and emotional stability. During this time, he changed his occupation from actor to social worker, reclaimed his Marrano heritage, committed himself to a spiritual path, and at the end of five years, entered into a serious, intimate, and long-lasting relationship.*

Why was Joel so successful in transforming his life? No doubt he was a resilient child.[4] He possessed a powerful creative imagination and a mentality that ceaselessly sought his own spiritual, psychological, and interpersonal development. He illustrates many characteristics that experts link with resilience; he is proactive, socially connected, self-disciplined, with the ability to organize, problem-solve, and persevere. How important was the unconditional acceptance and constancy provided in therapy?

Perhaps all of these factors contributed to his extraordinary transformation. However, the role of writing cannot be underestimated. I still have about 700 pages of e-mails that document Joel's emotional journey (yes, 700!). Even during periods of his life when he was not in therapy, writing in his journal functioned as a natural stabilizing agent following the turbulent seas of his childhood. The journal provided a place to dock that was a respite from the world. It gave Joel the opportunity to view the world from his own private observation deck. His reflections enabled him to envision and create the man he was going to become. Most important of all, Joel had a locus of control that helped him to come home to his truest, inviolable self—the journal that was an anchor.

~ 5 ~

Tír na mBan
(Gaelic for Land of Women)
Maryellen Bova

"Who, if I cried out, would hear me among the angels' hierarchies?"
(Rilke, The First Elegy).[1] There are said to be intermediaries between
earth and heaven—those known as angels, demons, gods and goddesses, but their visitations are rarely granted to mortals. However, when a
small, innocent child is pushed to her ultimate edge of being, physically
and emotionally, divine messengers from the heavens descend to help.

For the first few years of her life, Maryellen's grandmother provided
a soft haven for Maryellen and her siblings whenever she could. Her
grandmother, of Irish-Scottish background, showered Maryellen with
the Celtic stories and songs of her legacy. She also taught her to speak
in the ancient tongue. Is it any wonder that at moments when
Maryellen's life is threatened, the goddesses themselves intercede?

This is Maryellen's story.

The power of the crayon, the pencil, the marker, and the pen used to be my worst nemesis.

The first time I realized that I was different from other children was when I was in kindergarten and Mommy was called into school because I was not coloring correctly. I sat there feeling extremely stupid as Teacher explained to Mommy that I could not grasp the concept that I should color in pictures and not outside them. I disagreed. I did not want to color the body of Elephant or Girl. I liked them black and white and I put my colors around them so they would have good thoughts and days. I was creating a colorful world for them and no one else saw that.

"Are you retarded or just plain stupid? Everyone knows to color in the people. So, which is it—retarded or stupid?" asked Mommy as we walked out of school and headed toward home.

Her voice was angry and I knew that if if I did not give her an answer, there would be a slap in front of people before we reached the two blocks home, so I said, "Stupid."

"That's fucking right—you are stupid and don't you forget that!"

The next day I returned to kindergarten, faced with the dilemma of coloring in Monkey, and I cried. Teacher made me sit in the dark in the anteroom (the small room between classrooms) until I cried and begged to come out. I was only allowed out if I would color Monkey, and, as I colored Monkey, I cried and my tears fell upon the paper. I was violating Monkey's body, and I knew I would never want anyone to color on me.

The battle between Teacher and me continued as I broke all my crayons in half and was locked in the anteroom over and over again. Her cruelty toward me increased over the year, and Teacher would instantly lock me up in the anteroom if I hesitated for even a second before defiling Animals and People of my coloring book. And, when she called home about my problem, Mommy would slap me and shout, "Are you stupid or retarded?"

"Stupid," was the correct answer I would give, hanging my head down in shame. Mommy never asked why I did the things I did—I imagined she would ask me why I did not wish to color on the Animals or People. And, proudly, I would tell her, and she would realize that I was right, and she would stop slapping me . . . yelling at me—but that never happened.

Of course, as I progressed, the pencil soon caused me trouble in my writing abilities. In second grade, I was preparing to make Communion and we had to fill out a paper on how we would serve the Lord. I was so excited because I knew that I was picking the right job, so I spent lots of time neatly writing on my paper. My pencil felt so good in my hand as I wrote. One week later, when Sister handed back my paper, there was a large red zero and one comment: RE-DO. Tears ran down my cheeks. Sister came to see why I was crying, and I said, "But this is how I want to serve the Lord."

"Maryellen, you cannot be a priest—girls are nuns."

"I don't want to be a nun," I cried.

"Why not?" Sister's red face leaned into me and the other kids looked away. "Women are nuns!"

"I want to be a priest and I can be good at it," I cried.

"Maryellen, you cannot . . . will not be a priest, and I advise you to stop that nonsense now," Sister said as she moved in closer to my face.

"No," I said.

The smack across my face came so quickly that my head jerked back and my words hung in my throat, silenced.

"If I hear one more word about this nonsense, I will send you to the Monsignor! Do you understand?" Sister said loud enough for all the kids to hear.

The Monsignor was scary, and no one ever went to the Monsignor and lived to tell about it—that was what I had heard.

Sister pulled her face back, snatched my paper off my desk and proceeded to rip it up. The kids looked at me and then away as Sister walked back to the front and threw my words in the garbage.

When I went home, Mommy was there with a slap and, "Are you stupid or retarded?"

"Stupid."

I didn't tell Mommy that, in my imagination, I was a priest. I didn't tell her about the women who came and visited me. I didn't tell her how they would tell me that I was smart.

Cliodna was my best friend, and she looked like me, but she was smarter than I was and she usually knew the answers. Rhiannon, who looked like a beautiful Mommy, was very sweet to me and she would sing songs to me when I was upset or when my bed moved up and down in the middle of the night. She was the one with Cliodna, who would tell me to lie in the bed of roses until the bed stopped moving and Daddy would go back to his bed. Danu, who looked just like my Grandma, would hide in the ceiling to make sure no one slipped into the bathroom while I bathed, and she would tell me if Daddy was coming.

In fourth grade, I discovered the Goddess Medusa. I was at the Parkchester Library doing research on mythology, and I found Medusa, or, rather she found me. I read about how Medusa meant female wisdom. She was the keeper of the feminine mask, which was used to guard and protect women and the secret knowledge of the Divine Feminine. Her mask served as a warning to men that they should keep away!

Medusa lived in a sacred grove with priestesses and protected women. She was once very beautiful, and then the men in society set out to destroy her. Images of her beautiful face appeared in all of the books I pulled from the shelf, but there were also the snakehead demonic images, which did not scare me.

I read how Zeus raped Metis and then swallowed her up. Because Metis was so great in her wisdom, Zeus's head became pregnant, and Athena was born from the top of his skull. Zeus stole Metis's body by raping her and then stole her wisdom by swallowing her. Athena was born out of the violence and destruction of another goddess. I was frightened that Daddy would eat me up.

As I spent the afternoon and the evening in that library, I learned that Athena was not very nice. Medusa, the beautiful goddess, who protected women with her mask, was loved by many, and Athena was jealous of her. One day, while Medusa was worshipping in Athena's temple, Poseidon raped Medusa. Athena was so outraged at Medusa for the act that she decided to punish Medusa by turning her into a snake-haired creature.

Medusa's voice was silenced, and the only power she now possessed was the power to turn men to stone. I was unhappy about her voice being silenced, but I wished for the secret power of turning men into stone. It was really sad that Athena helped Perseus in his quest to cut off Medusa's head with a sickle. I prayed that I could become Medusa, before her head was cut off, and turn Daddy into stone.

Soon Medusa became part of my Goddess world and our field of roses, and she joined Cliodna, Rhiannon, and Danu. Sometimes she was her really pretty self, and then, other times, when I really needed her, she had the snakes ready to attack. I felt safe to have her with me. Sometimes I would tell the kids on the playground that I was Medusa and that I could turn them to stone by looking them in the eye. That kept them from hitting me or calling me names, and I enjoyed the power that gave me; however, I still was unable to turn Daddy into stone.

In fifth grade art class, we were instructed to draw a self-portrait, and I was so excited about the colors of my markers and paints. I made yellow and orange snakes coming out of my red hair. I shaped my eyes perfectly round with red and black pupils that held rocks within. My body was colored black with red drops everywhere. I was really proud, until Teacher called home.

"What the fuck is wrong with you? Are you fucking stupid or retarded?" Mommy shouted at me as Daddy stared at the floor.

I wondered if Medusa could turn women into stone as I watched Mommy move her arms around, screaming. I prayed for snakes to roar and hiss from my head and then I would look at her . . . but Medusa did not come as Mommy reached over and slapped my face.

"Are you fucking stupid or retarded?" she spat at me. I hated her at that moment. I hated Daddy for staring at the floor.

"Neither!" I shouted back, and Mommy punched me across the face. I fell to the floor and stared at her through blurry, tearful eyes, the taste of blood on my lips.

"What are you? Stupid or fucking retarded?" Mommy screamed as she kicked my legs.

"I am Maryellen," I said softly, looking to Daddy for help, but his eyes were glued to the floor, and I hoped he would go blind.

"What a fucking joke! Did you hear that, Bill—she knows her name!

What do you think of that?"

Daddy kept looking at that floor, and I hoped it would open up and he would fall through.

"You are not Maryellen! You are fucking stupid! Retarded! And a fucking nobody—got that? Got that, you fucking little idiot?" Mommy kicked me in my ribs, again and again.

I winced in pain and said, "Yes, Mommy."

"Yes, what?"

"Yes, Mommy, I got it."

"You got that you are a fucking, stupid nobody, right?"

"Yes, Mommy, I am stupid."

"Good, now get the fuck out of my sight."

I pulled myself up and went to my room, and there was Danu, Rhiannon, and Cliodna waiting to comfort me as I cried into my pillow. That night, Medusa came to me while I slept. Daddy did not come into my room that night.

After that, I hated art and decided never to draw or paint anything again. And when Teacher would call home, I would tell Mommy I was too stupid to draw or paint, and she would not bother me at all. Being stupid was good enough for Mommy.

Of course, the pen would betray me once again. In junior high, we were assigned to write a poem about obedience. It had something to do with some essay on Civil Disobedience and this was Teacher's creative way of responding.

I went home to my room, ignoring Brother's and Sister's request to play wall ball, excited about writing poetry, and wrote about my obedience.

Daddy Said
Daddy said
I was a very obedient girl

and

sometimes

his pillow
would smother
my face

to help me
remember

to obey
and surrender

When I finished writing the poem, I knew I could never give it to Teacher because she would call Mommy, and I would be on the floor saying, "Stupid." So, I hid that poem away in the back of my dresser, forgot about it, and wrote a lame poem about dogs and obedience. I didn't get a good grade, but I also didn't get a slap or a punch.

That was short lived. A few weeks later, Mommy went through my bureau and found the poem. She was waiting for me, sitting at the kitchen table, as I walked through the door, and I could sense her mood was foul. Brother and Sister were called from their rooms and told to go play outside. They both looked at me as though my death was about to occur, and Brother had tears in his eyes. Sister said bye as she walked out with Brother.

Mommy stared at me, and I was afraid.

"What's the matter?" I asked, swallowing.

"You think you are so fucking smart, don't you?" her voice quivering as her fists clenched.

"No, I don't."

"Oh yes you do—the little fucking nobody thinks she's a genius, but she's a fucking stupid cunt!" she screamed and lunged at me, fists flying.

I remember kicks. Punches. Words thrown at me. I held myself in a fetal position trying to protect my face. She tore at my clothes. She tore at me. She punched and kicked until I passed out. When I awoke, the real terror began.

That night when Daddy came home, Mommy made me place a match to my poem.

I had to tell Daddy that I was sorry I had written a lie about him. I had to tell Mommy that I was sorry for acting like a temptress and thinking bad thoughts about Daddy.

The poem burned in the pot Daddy used for potatoes. Words flew at me as the flames grew and died out. Mommy, Daddy, and I stood there watching the paper disappear, and I wished I could too.

The last words before I went to bed without supper were from Mommy, "If you ever write another fucking word . . . I will fucking kill you! Do you hear that, you stupid, fucking, retarded nobody?"

"Yes, Mommy," I said, as I felt the flames devour my body. The goddesses around me sobbed. For once I closed them out . . . I wished we would all die.

Later that night, Danu told me how to hold the wet cloth. Cliodna held me in her arms and Rhiannon kissed my forehead. I prayed for Jesus to take me away. I promised Him I would be a good girl in Heaven. But, I guess, Jesus was too busy to hear my voice.

The next poem I wrote was about that day, but this time I hid the poem at school. I wrote that poem so I would believe—because the truth was too unbearable and no one would ever believe. Even I do not believe. I took all my dolls and threw them away. I buried all of them in the trash.

To this day, I still feel the scorching. The tears. I see the words flying at me—the whole heat of it lives, trapped within my soul and even when I put the pen to paper, it is smudged with ashes and smoldering in flames.

The Heat

She was playing with her friend
in a playroom. They were dressing
Ken and Barbie. She was nine. Her friend
was more advanced and knew a way that the dolls
could have more fun. Her friend said there were sins
growing inside of them and they hadn't a choice. Her friend
traced Ken's body with a finger, stopped at his pants, turned his
head backwards, struck the matchbox, and his body slowly melted in the heat.

Mommy told me this as though it would explain everything.

She brought the memories to me of the heat. She carried them
underneath her breath. She gave them to me—in the mirrorless
walls, in the form of a glance, a scream in the night
as Daddy entered. In the way she told me
to cover my body, my growing body.
In the way she told me my body
was dirty and my mind
even worse when I
closed a door.
In the way
Mommy
held the
flame
to my
vagina
so that
she
might
melt
away
the
sins.

This is when I started to refer to Mommy as Athena. Like Medusa, I had been violated, and Mommy decided to punish me. Mommy was Athena, the warrior goddess, who helped men defeat women. I never called her Athena to her face, but, in my mind, I shouted, Athena, Athena, oh you bitch!

She could turn me into an ugly creature, but she could not break me. I, like Medusa, still had some power, and I would turn men into stone. When Daddy came into my room, I fought hard and I know Athena heard my muffled cries from under the pillow over my face.

In the second week of ninth grade, September 1980, at 6:00 a.m., I set off to work—the same stupid job I had for the past two years. Brother and I delivered newspapers to over 100 people every morning. We would do the first three blocks together, each taking a side of the apartment buildings, until we got to the fourth block and then, Brother would hit Beach and I would stay on Thieriot. I remember stepping into my last building and being excited about nearly being done with this crap. I hated delivering newspapers. I hated the black filthy ink on my hands, I hated putting together the Sunday papers, I hated carrying the weight of all those papers, but we needed the money. Daddy had been sick and having a hard time at work and Athena was not making enough money, so Brother and I had to help out.

As I stepped into that last building, I hit the elevator button and then heard the pounding footsteps racing toward me. I turned around just as Man grabbed my arm. In his other hand, Man held a knife and pressed it against my cheek. The knife came back with my blood, and Man licked the knife. I froze. In the distance, I heard Rhiannon screaming to run, but I could not move. Cliodna was telling me to breathe, but my blood was on the tongue of Man and then the elevator doors opened and he pushed me in.

Man took me to the roof. We were there for a long time, and I remember Cliodna crying a lot. The sun beat down on me and the tar and the tiny pebbles dug into my back. Rhiannon kept telling me to come lie in the field of roses, but, every time I tried, Man would hurt me harder. He wanted me to be with him fully and every time I slipped away, Man hurt me more. Danu sang to me those Gaelic songs my grandmother once sang and I tried to lose myself in those melodies. When I thought it was all over, Man told me to stand.

"Do you want to be a fucking nun?" Man shouted.

"No," I said.

"You want to be a fucking nun—all you Irish girls want to be fucking nuns!"

"But I don't want to be," I said, which I really meant, but, somehow, this was a trick question. I just knew it.

I heard the pigeons on the roof floor, and I looked away. The pain hit me hard in my neck as the knife came across. Again. And again. Man and Perseus on their quest, attempting to behead me. The knife moved in and out of my body. In my stomach . . . out. In my chest . . . out. In my face . . . out. In my back . . . out. I fell to the floor. Kicks to my head. Kicks to my ribs. Rhiannon shouting to hold on. I blacked out as the last kick hit me in the side of my face, and something in my head exploded.

I awoke, in the hospital, days later to Mommy standing over me. I could not swallow. My voice had been silenced. I had a tracheotomy in my throat, they told me later. Mommy stared at me. I could not speak. Tears flowed from my eyes.

"You're okay," Mommy said, "You're going to be just fine."

I looked up at her, and, for a moment, I believed she cared.

"Don't tell anyone you were raped—they will think you're dirty, and Daddy and I don't want people to believe that. Tell them he tried, but you fought him off . . ."

What she said after that didn't matter. Athena, Athena, oh you bitch!

For a while after that, I spoke nothing, wrote nothing. I stayed in my world with Medusa, who was finally able to help me turn men into stone—Daddy never touched me again. He still looked at me . . . that made me sick. Rhiannon held me in her arms and sang songs with Danu. They both tucked me into bed. And Cliodna rested by my side day and night. I remained locked in my sacred grove where Medusa once lived.

In my sacred grove, where my voice had been cut, I screamed. I colored the outside of Animals and People. I never touched their bodies, defiled them with what I believed should be their color. I was head Goddess. Medusa, Rhiannon, Danu and Cliodna listened to me. I drew myself with snakeheads and evil eyes, and Men stayed away from me. I chanted poems about pillows, obedience, the heat, the knife, the blood on Man's tongue, and I screamed: Athena, Athena, oh you bitch!

I wasn't stupid. I was that girl to whom bad things had happened. What people didn't know was that I was that girl to whom bad things happened before the knife and the blood entered my life. I was the nobody everybody failed to notice. And now, here's my story. The power of the pen has brought me pain and tears, but now it brings me strength and tears.

The story that you have just read may seem surrealistic, abstract, or unreal. However, it is a true story, bearing witness to senseless violence.[2] It is a story of abuse, a story as old as time itself, unique only because of the extreme degree of violence and Maryellen's ability to tell us about it. Maryellen has taken us back in time (time-shifting), as she relives experiences that occurred to the wounded child who lives within her. In cases of severe abuse, when pain is more than can be borne, it is not uncommon for a person to have out-of-the-body experiences, during which awareness is split off, and a temporary trance-like state offers escape from the pain.

The theologian might say that Maryellen experienced spiritual visions. The psychologist may argue that these trances are "dissociation."[3] Yeats, William Blake, Garcia Lorca, and other poets might protest that when life itself is at risk and the self pushes against its own limits, demons and angels, gods and goddesses unleash the creative imagination.[4]

The ancient stories of mythology come out of the oral tradition of storytelling. Storytelling was borne out of our need to understand ourselves, others, and our connection to a spiritual power greater than our own. The mythological figures are appealing because, despite their divinity, they are subject to the same passions, temptations, and errors as humans. Athena, Zeus, and Medusa are mythological beings who aptly serve to mirror the violence and usurping of personal power that Maryellen experiences.

The magic of the poetic employs the archetypes as metaphors. In a marvelous maneuver of creative defensive coping, the mind offers the figures of Rhiannon, Danu and Cliodna, the Celtic goddesses, as touchstones of safety during imperiled moments. These goddesses are more than literary devices. They are the personifications of the kindness, love, and support given in early childhood by Maryellen's grandmother. They provide a meaningful framework for Maryellen's experience, a glimmering of understanding and hope in a childhood that is bleak and painful.

Although punished early on for her observations of reality, Maryellen perseveres with her crayons, markers, and pens. These are tools of empowerment, providing stolen moments of freedom of expression in a house of abuse. At age twelve, when her mother burns her writing and warns her that she will kill her if she writes again, Maryellen's true voice is stifled. Later, at age fourteen, surviving a brutal rape when left for dead, her voicebox sustains multiple knife wounds. She writes, "In my sacred grove, where my voice had been cut, I screamed. I colored. Outside of Animals and People. I never touched their bodies." Note how Maryellen immediately exits the real world and enters the safehouse of the creative imagination. "The sacred grove" is a place where violation cannot take place. Maryellen refuses to take the perpetrator's role. Instead, she is careful not to violate the boundaries of animals or people.

After many months, Maryellen regains use of her voice. In the years that follow, she reclaims her voice in another way—through the ritual of writing. In over thirty journals, she has written black and white testimony of her life experiences. Writing is a process that provides unique properties for trauma survivors. When capturing large feelings with small black squiggles, a sense of mastery prevails. Although writing is a dialogue with oneself, the writer is both the creator and the audience. Different parts of the self have the opportunity for expression. When trauma has taken place, the reader may view the events like a spectator watching a trial. Maryellen as reader may serve as a mediator to help her to process and integrate everything that has happened.

The writer who is reading her own work is ultimately strengthened in self-awareness. This self-awareness, made possible by the observing ego, naturally moves the writer toward reflection, analysis and progression of thought, making transformation possible. Dr. David Johnson, co-director of the New Haven Center of Post-Traumatic Stress, writes, "If the moment of trauma is fundamentally an act of destruction, then writing serves, symbolically as a restitutive act of creation. To victims of trauma, the act of writing calls forth the realization, 'I exist; I am not gone.' Once written, the piece acquires its own autonomy; it is no longer in the victim. Writing is a birth."[5] Despite severe abuse, rape, and eleven stabbings to the neck, face, chest, stomach, back and head, the creative, spiritual self cannot be destroyed; it is resourceful, generative, and resilient.

Today Maryellen lives with her husband and four sons in upstate New York. She is a teacher of high-school English and encourages young people to express their true selves through writing. Dubbed the "Goddess Coach," Maryellen also facilitates empowerment workshops for women to help them make contact with the Divine Feminine that lies within. Rhiannon, Cliodna, Danu, and Medusa have never abandoned her.

~ 6 ~

The Poem That Was a Prayer
Sister Mary Sullivan

"If you have fear, you cannot have faith, and if you have faith, you cannot have fear." This is a popular saying in the church. But does faith actually preclude fear? Sister Mary Sullivan has committed herself to a life of service in the church since the age of twenty-one. At age sixty-seven, Sister Mary is diagnosed with a tumor, and despite her faith in the Divine, copes with a terror that is all too human. She is told she needs a dangerous operation that may leave her blind or disabled if she survives. Sister Mary is the last surviving member of her immediate family. Who will be there for her? And what of God? Will He be there for her?

Sister Mary's story is about a health crisis, but it is also the story of a girl in search of her father, and a mature woman in search of God. Fear, doubt, and anger would be natural expressions for anyone in Sister Mary's situation. However, Sister Mary, a woman of faith, has been taught to "turn the other cheek." Where can she go to express her feelings?

This is Sister Mary's story.

THE EARLY YEARS

Eager for scraps of my father, I have stood a beggar at the threshold of others' memories. Dad died sixty-six years ago. I was four; my brother Joe, ten; my brother Ted, nine. I was introduced to abandonment at a tender age, and periodically through my life, this demon has reappeared and tormented me through different experiences. But my story is not a sad one. My family, though diminished by Dad's death, was strong and joyful; we were always there for one another.

My mother and father were English teachers. The library was my favorite room in the house where I grew up. The library's shelves were crammed with books. One particular bookcase was devoted to nothing but "The Harvard Classics." Dad had gone to Harvard and graduated in 1920. I knew if I could but read those books and understand them I would somehow be connected with Dad.

Early on I intuited the ability to read and comprehend what I had read as "power." My two siblings, whom I adored, read, and I wanted to catch up with them. At the age of six, my mother brought me to a local branch of the main library in Trenton, New Jersey. It was two miles from home. Mom showed me how to walk there—cross the railroad tracks, span the bridge over the canal, and stop on the way for a brief visit in our local parish church, Blessed Sacrament.

I received my first library card. Exhilarated and heady with freedom, I began a love affair with books. I could only take out four books at a time. In the space of a day I would complete my reading and go back for more. I graduated to taking the bus to downtown Trenton, and, armed with Mom's, Joe's, and Ted's library cards, I would take out sixteen books. Once a week I headed to the main library and got my fix.

I started to write my own books by the time I was eight. My Mother discovered the most effective punishment was not to allow me to read. Bereft of library books and the comics, I turned to writing on my own. She could not deprive me of what I myself had written. I wrote and rewrote the same story. I called the book *Diamond Harbor*. My first chapter, "The Linden

Tree," was always the same. It featured a widower who had four sons and one daughter. Freudian, eh? I killed off my mother, multiplied the number of brothers, and I was the center of attention!

In our family library sat a big comfortable chair. Mom called it "Dad's chair."

Whenever we were afraid or needed a solution to a problem my mother would invite us to sit in that chair and, "Talk it over with your Dad." As Roman Catholics we believe in a religious tenet called the "Communion of the Saints." Without realizing it, we three youngsters were receiving our first education in how to pray. Our prayer was conversational and spoken out of need. We trusted in a father (God? Dad?) who loved us, protected us, and wanted what was best for us. Prayer became habitual; it was non-threatening, and took place in the room of books. Books, prayer, God as Father, my Dad were all one great big wonderful mélange that comforted me, set me free, and gave me a place to go whenever I was in need.

COMMUNICATOR AND FAMILY HISTORIAN

I entered religious life straight out of college. I was twenty-one. I am now seventy. My dad died at forty-three of colon cancer, Mom at seventy-three of lung cancer and emphysema, Ted at sixty-seven of lung cancer and emphysema, and Joe, the day after his seventy-first birthday, of emphysema. I thought my father's death when I was four was traumatic for me. I have since discovered that the loss of my siblings has been even more heart wrenching.

Now I am the only depository of the family stories, the only one left of this generation, and the oldest person alive in the family tree. It is I who am called upon to fill in the gaps of health, of immigration, of where and how the family lived, worked, fought and loved. Here is an excerpt of my six page poem, "Teapots and Soup Tureens," expressing my feelings about family.

I hold a soup tureen with reverence, respect, awe
It holds the soup
The soup I call New England Clam Chowder
A soup rich in cream, butter, clams, onions, salt, pepper, broth, potatoes
My origins are Irish; a famine starved people who survived on potatoes
My American roots are from New England; a briny rich people . . .

The most recent death in the Sullivan family (who will tell his story?)
spurs me on, urges me, compels me
to stir the chowder
to taste the separate components
to acknowledge that it is not chowder without all the ingredients
  rich cream of ancestors
  sweet butter of love
  tough clams of resilience
  feisty onions that add bitterness and character to the mix
  salt of tears
  pepper of disagreements
  briny broth of experience of staying together
  potatoes, starchy substance of everyday living
  the bit of bacon to enhance its Irish flavor

I stir
savor the fragrant steam
rejoice that it is my soup
my homemade Sullivan recipe
I need to claim all of our soup
the genetic inheritance of depression
the genetic inheritance of alcoholism
the dark side of anger, resentment, unresolved, unwanted relationships
the untold, and therefore unheard stories

It is time to reopen the recipe book
It is time to stop the chowder from burning

It is time to scrape the bottom of the pot
It is time . . .
to remember the stories
to tell the stories
to share my parents' generation's stories
to share Joe's, Ted's and my generation's stories
to gather the laughter and tears of this family
to ladle out the sweet saltiness of this chowder
for the stories are my progeny . . .

I am that soup tureen
two handled
ceramic
fat, ponderous
vulnerable to breakage
with a ladle that is long and deep, reaching back into family history
May I scoop out the soup
laugh and cry with the spillage
and say, "Come and eat. Here is the Sullivan Family Chowder
There is no other like it. I am proud of that."

I had trained to be a speech therapist and majored in communications in college. I was noted in my province as a "good communicator." I was trained to facilitate religious retreats and did so in the United States, Holland, Ireland, and England. In 1996, I was asked by my congregation, Our Lady of the Retreat in the Cenacle, to live with our Cenacle Sisters in the Philippines. I was asked to acculturate and share with our North American sisters what the experience had been like for me. I began to write seriously and found enjoyment there in a new and different way.

I trudged all over the Philippines with my dictionary and thesaurus and writing pad. I did what we call "Theological Reflection." That is to say, what I experienced personally was brought before my God, reflected on, and refracted back to others in terms of spiritual essays. Poetry was a short cut to my heart and my feelings. I found that I could not live without my dictionary, my thesaurus, and my bible in just that precise order. On a feeling level, I note that, when I write, I never feel hungry (I am a compulsive eater). I lose all sense of time. I feel filled, sated, satisfied. Energy courses through me. It is only in the written word that I am simultaneously free and at home.

CRISIS

In 2002 I was diagnosed with a tumor on my pituitary gland. This tumor was in a precarious position; if I survived the operation, I could lose my sight or hearing. I was not afraid of death, but I was terrified that I might be left disabled. In the same week that I received this news, I was scheduled to attend a poetry workshop with John Fox. Unbeknownst to me, God had provided an avenue for me to release my feelings.

Two poems came easily on the first day of the workshop. One addressed my sadness, and the other addressed my fear.

What Could I Do but Stay
Vesper still
The porch calls me to prayer
I praise the sky with my eyes
Turn to go in
My hand lingers on the doorknob
I hesitate
Once again I lean into the darkness
Look outwards, upwards
Last moonrise?
Last time to witness the stars' dance?
What could I do but stay?

Insomnia

Fear and terror litter the floor
poke up through the mattress
punch
provoke
probe
Sleep, their ransom's demand I pay
All night
I press, press, press down
At dawn's light
I see the demons still
unmoved
unappeased
ready to pounce when next darkness falls

I continued to name and claim the tumor through my writing. It helped to absorb my shock and at the same time, brought me closer to owning this dilemma.

Visitor

My tumor announced its arrival last Monday
It journeyed incrementally
Trekked inexorably
Usurped space
Demanded attention
Bestowed terror
Laughed in my face
I want to claim
Sunday
The day before Monday
The heat and humidity I complained about
That was the day I didn't know
the tumor's tendrils

already encroached
already rooted
already displaced
the joy of taking out the garbage
of seeing the clouds choke the moon
of smelling moist earth, linden trees and acrid green scat.

The workshop ended. I knew I was in big trouble. I needed to talk this out with someone, a skilled professional. I called chaplains at hospitals and asked if they knew a health-care professional who would be with me to address my fears and cope with the decisions I had to make. They kept recommending me to spiritual directors. I did not want a spiritual director. I was adamant about that. This situation went beyond my role as a nun. It was about being broken and being human. There is a saying in the church, "If you have fear, you cannot have faith, and if you have faith, you cannot have fear." I needed to explore the territory of this frightening journey, and I wanted no judgment in the process.

POETIC MEDICINE

I decided I wanted to write my way through this. I turned to the Internet. The National Association for Poetry Therapy list of poetry therapists yielded the name and number of Dr. Sherry Reiter, a clinical social worker and registered poetry therapist in New York. She asked how I would feel working with a non-Catholic or whether I might prefer someone of my own faith. Ironically, the fact that she was of a different faith served to free me. Most Catholics cannot tolerate fear in a sister. They find faith and fear incompatible; this shuts off any real communication. Without knowing it, I had chosen an observant Jew. It was September, and our sessions were scheduled not to interfere with the holidays. Knowing that my therapist was religiously observant was somehow comforting. Dr. Reiter gave me permission to be myself; I could be totally free and truthful.

Because I could not travel, we scheduled hour-long phone conversations. My therapist would suggest themes to write on. I would e-mail my poems to her prior to the session. When I began therapy, I was in a state of tension and panic. It was hard to sleep. My first assignment was to find a poem that gave me comfort. I was to memorize it, and say it continually throughout my day whenever I felt afraid, as well as before going to sleep. I knew instantly what poem I would choose. It was "Let Evening Come" by Jane Kenyon. I typed it up and carried the paper everywhere with me. It builds to the final stanza: "Let it come, as it will, and don't be afraid. / God does not leave us / comfortless, so let evening come."

At this time, I was painfully aware of the tumor entwined around my nasal cavity that threatened to destroy my ability to see, to hear, and to smell. Visiting a farmer's market became the inspiration for the following poem:

Deep Well Material

Fridays
July through October,
our town hosts
local Jersey farmers.

Harvest heaps
jostle, crowd each other;
vie for room
on the display tables;
vendors on one side,
customers, the other.

Cerulean blue plums,
magenta skinned eggplant,
bright red, dark green peppers,
blueberries, strawberries, blackberries,
yellow squash, brown flecked golden pears,

dusty blue grapes,
corpulent beefsteak tomatoes, heavy in my hands,
rouge tinted peaches, fuzzy to my touch,
fragrant basil, pungent scallions, nose arresting mint.

Sweet white corn demands its own table,
four-sided, available to all.
Like a medieval town's well
gossip, information, pleasantries
easily exchanged.

September corn,
past prime ripened.
I strip one
face dry wizened kernels. Today, Friday,
two women stand next to me,
their conversation loud
almost cell phone intrusive
to my ears.

"He's getting worse. He hides money and accuses me of stealing it. An MIT graduate and he can't even make out a bank deposit slip any longer."

"That's the way it was with my Harry."

I shuck another ear of corn.
Dark worms uncurl
before my eyes.
Ugh!

"That's the trouble with head tumors. It just gets worse and they don't see it. They
think they're functioning and they're not."

More worms,
dehydrated kernels.
I strip; cast aside
find a good ear
and save it.

"What makes it worse I see friends on the street. They turn around and walk away
from me. They must think it's contagious."

I, who was just told I have a tumor
growing in my head;
its tentacles stretch, invade
my optic nerve, sinus cavity.

I cannot shuck this conversation.
I attempt to strip the resonance of words
curling and unfurling like worms
in my ears.

The colors of life spill over the tables.
I face my own September prime.
Will I know my own deterioration?
Do I want to know?

Only after writing this did I realize that the tumor, like the vegetables in the poem, was crowding out everything else in my life now. I was encompassed with the tumor as it jostled and vied for my attention. My therapist invited me to dialogue with the tumor. I wrote:

Tumor, you are you
Tumor, I am I
Tumor, I cannot allow you to define me.

Our boundaries had somehow merged. Surgery would provide the total separation, but in the meantime I was delineating my boundaries.

My next assignment was to explore my relationship with God through writing. We were, in a sense, like dance partners but I was stumbling on the dance floor. I went through feelings of fear, bargaining, and reluctant submission. One of the poems I wrote was called "The Dance."

This tight Irish body
finds it hard to dance

I took tap
I took ballet
Dance never took me

With God as partner
I attempt
a progressive two step

Why struggle?
Why not trust?
Dance, Mary,
Damn it; Dance
Surrender
Let God take the lead

During this period of time, I had a nightmare that repeated itself again and again with slight variations. It was a dream in which I must traverse a suspension bridge overlooking deep water.

The Nightmare

Again
Again
And again
Always again
The same dream

The nightmare starts with
a long, long entrance
to a suspension bridge

I feel my stomach drop
Butterflies flutter
try to escape my body
I attempt to free myself
from a drive
I know
has no escape . . .
I see plainly
the bridge
the span
the height
the water underneath . . .
I am full of fear
for my gaze sees clearly what I
must traverse
I never see the land from which I depart
I never see my arrival point
I never see other cars, other travelers

I walk across a wide bridge
with open grids
I can look down, through
to the water directly below

I enter the vestibule
of an elevator
When the doors automatically close
the vestibule gives way
to a glass room
I ride; I rise
I see below
a long, long way
The butterflies beat inside, unable to extricate themselves

My fear tells me I am angry
But of what?
But of whom?

The journey?
The length?
The impotence?
The unknown?
The aloneness?
The damn ineluctable force?

I dread sleep

Again
Again
And again
Always again
The same dream

I cannot escape the journey
I cannot escape the dream
I cannot escape the anger
I cannot escape the fear
I cannot escape the operation on the tumor in my head

Nightmare

My dialogues with God continued. Dr. Reiter urged me to be unafraid of expressing my anger and fear directly to God. While such dialogue was in the tradition of Tevye, from *Fiddler on the Roof*, it was also reminiscent of my childhood, sitting in my father's chair unburdening my heart.

I entitled this next poem "Tenebrae." It is a name we especially apply to the prayers of Holy Week said together in worship. The church is in darkness with only a few flickering candles to give light to the words we recite. It is the time when Jesus is facing his own death; He struggles with his own fears of the suffering that lies before him. He trusts his Father and surrenders the future to Him. I was being asked to do the same. My poem suggests my own struggle to surrender to a God whom I trust and I know loves me.

Tenebrae

I love my words
substantive
succulent
opulent
mellifluous
image evocative
lodestars of meaning
rip tide dangerous

I fall into night
opaque
starless
no compass of words to guide me

Now it is God
Who undertows
lures
draws
pulls

125

me into my own personal Tenebrae
the psalmody of night
the prayer of Holy Week

Before my God
I lie prostrate
silent
visionless
quiescent
aware, oh so aware,
that it is a time to be led
led into the event, into the process
by a Father whom I believe
loves me

Faith lies under tiers
(under tears)
of doubt, distrust, discouragement
I cannot see
I need to take the hand
of a God Who sees
I need to wade with unhesitating trust
into this sea of darkness.

THE BREAKTHROUGH POEM

About a week before the operation, I wrote what I think of as my most significant breakthrough poem. It is entitled "Soundings." Not so long ago, before sonar was used to measure the depth of water, a line of rope with knots was lowered into the water to sound and mark its depths.[1] "Running out of line" signifies deep water and a clear path.

Soundings
God sounds out my soul
tosses down a line
measures the depth of my faith
How far down before bottom reached
Are there fathoms enough to carry me to shore
Will I capsize
I snivel fear
cast a line up
into the heart of God
trust with invincible hope
I will run out of line.

All six weeks of laborious writing brought me to this moment. This was it. It was the peak, the crown of all my tears, struggles, fears, and words. Upon hearing this poem, my poetry therapist said, "Now this is your comfort poem. Memorize it. Take it with you everywhere. As they wheel you into the operating room, recite the words. As you wake from anesthesia, have the words on your lips."

And I did. It truly became my comfort poem. No one had ever suggested that I memorize my own words. A tremendous sense of power was awakened in me by my own words. It was my mantra. It was my prayer.

I survived the operation. The tumor was benign. I recuperated with no impairments from the surgery. That December, my Christmas message was a copy of *Soundings* and the following:

A year of struggle, surrender, and surgery has taught me:
Christmas coaxes Calvary
past death;
promises Resurrection;
posits
Love's legacy, Life
Longing for Life runs rampant through my heart.

127

May it do so in yours.

Sister Mary shows exceptional courage in discarding the persona of the strong and never-doubting nun to seek the help that she needs, even though it is outside the confines of the church. She follows her instincts successfully. She needs to express her feelings, and be "in all her brokenness." Sister Mary is blessed with a love of writing, as well as a disciplined nature. As the poetry therapist, I serve as a guide and companion through this crisis. However, Sister Mary's psychological transformation is informed primarily by the wisdom of her own writing experiences. These experiences are catalysts of the natural healing process.

First and foremost, Sister Mary writes for self-regulation of emotion through containment and catharsis. Writing serves as a container to hold a kaleidoscope of feelings. Distance is needed from the onslaught of terror. She is able to draw boundaries around her fear, to separate the tumor, her disease, from herself, and to contain the excessive emotion. "Tumor, you are you / Tumor, I am I / Tumor, I cannot let you define me." By shifting time, space, and matter in her writing, Sister Mary achieves the necessary distance for coping. The process of writing serves several purposes. Externalizing this crisis in words makes it available for reflection, witnessing, and problem solving. Because fear and anger tend to create disorder and chaos, Sister Mary is also writing for clarity and organization. Spiritually torn, it is important to dialogue with God; Sister Mary had been meditating, praying, and writing for many years before this crisis. Now, confused with anger and grief, Sister Mary continues to write to connect to the Divine.

In order to treat her insomnia, I suggest prescription poetry, the repetition of a peaceful poem to be said aloud prior to going to sleep as many times as necessary. Sister Mary's choice is Jane Kenyon's poem "Let Evening Come," and it is successful in helping her to relax. It is a unit of energy, spiritual, emotional, and cognitive, imported and embraced by her open mind, open heart, and open spirit; Eli Greifer would have called it a "psychograft - a transfusion of the soul."[2]

Eli Greifer was a pioneer in the field of poetry therapy who in the

1920s through the 1960s advocated memorizing inspirational poetry for a kind of "bloodless psychosurgery." The client is actually borrowing ego-strength from the poet. In Greifer's words, "We have here no less than a psychograft-by-memorization in the inmost reaches of the brain, where the soul can allow the soul-stuff of stalwart poet-prophets to 'take' and to become one with the spirit of the patient."[3] The poetry therapist may import a poem (bring in a published poem) or export a poem (bring out a poem from inside the client). Sister Mary benefits from both methods.

In fact, Sister Mary had her own personal code of significant symbols that were repeated throughout her poetry. The metaphor of water, "rip-tide dangerous," serves to further encapsulate her terror and anger. In one of the first poems, "Nightmare," Sister Mary looks over a terrifying expanse of water. In a later poem, Sister Mary refers to her terror as a "sea of darkness," as she wrestled with her faith: "Faith lies under tiers / (under tears) / of doubt, distrust, discouragement / I cannot see / I need to take the hand / of a God Who sees / I need to wade with unhesitating trust / into this sea of darkness." The health crisis is not only a crisis of the body; it is also a crisis of the soul.

Several weeks later, just prior to the operation, Sister Mary writes her breakthrough poem, "Soundings," in which water is central. However, the symbolism has changed; Sister Mary is the boat, and the sea of darkness has transformed into a sea of God's love. "(I) cast a line up / into the heart of God / trust with invincible hope / I will run out of line." Sister Mary transforms the depths of her fear into faith, tossing her line into the immeasurable sea of God's love. Ultimately Sister Mary's connection to God is reaffirmed and her zeal for life renewed.

Sometimes a poem is like a message in a bottle sent into the great ocean. We hope that it will be received on another shore, and we will be understood. Sometimes a poem is a question. Sometimes it is a declaration, a protest, or an apology. And as Sister Mary can attest, sometimes a poem is a prayer.

129

~ 7 ~

The Woman Who Went Night Fishing

Nadia Antonopoulos

Nadia's story is about a young girl on the verge of womanhood. Her feminine powers are still a mystery. Although she recognizes that sexuality is a powerful force, she is not prepared to deal with its consequences. Nadia is raised in a culture that encourages male dominance and female subservience. As a child, being the apple of her father's eye, Nadia's love bucket is filled by his attentiveness. However, with the approach of puberty, Dad retreats from his sensuous daughter, and her love bucket is now empty. How does a female get the attention and love she craves?

This is Nadia's story.

THE EARLY YEARS

All my life I thought there was something wrong with me. I am able to trace this feeling back to the age of three. During the day, Grandma took care of me and my cousin Nikos. She was a pious

Greek Orthodox woman, who often scolded us about our two options in life; there was heaven and there was hell. She often reminded me that I was evil, and there was a place in hell waiting for me. On the other hand, my cousin Nikos could do no wrong. She would lovingly watch Nikos and coax him to eat and dress, while I was, for the most part, ignored day after day.

Why was I less important than my cousin? What did he have that I didn't have? I ran as quickly as he did, made drawings just as pretty, and even spoke two languages (Greek and English), whereas he spoke only English. I decided that it must be his penis. Surely that was where his power came from. I wanted one desperately. And if I couldn't have a penis, I figured maybe wearing boy's clothes would do the trick. So every morning, I insisted that Nikos take off his clothes, and we swapped outfits. He was astonishingly passive and did as I commanded. Of course my mother would usually catch us before she left for work, and Nikos had to return my pretty dress to me. "Again?" my mother would say, "You always want whatever he has."

What I wanted, of course, was to be fussed over and loved.

I was sitting on the stoop with my cousin Nikos one day, furious with the injustice of my situation. A great anger swept over me. Impulsively I shoved Nikos, who fell wailing to the street below. Grandma was beside herself with anger. She screamed bloody murder as the swelling on Nikos' head rose to be the size of a giant egg. I was the Evil One. She let go of a stream of invectives, punctuated by "Githuta!" (Ass!)

I ran upstairs with stormy tears and spent most of the afternoon in my room. When my parents came home, I came downstairs. Pointing my finger at my Grandmother, I said, "You—You are the jackass!" It was confirmed —by the age of three, I knew I was going to Hell.

Thus, the demons of powerlessness and inferiority made themselves known to me at a very early age. Seeds of shame and guilt were planted at the same time. In the years that followed, I was to learn what it meant to be female in a Greek Orthodox family. There was a hard-clad hierarchy of power in Greek Orthodox culture and religion. My father's mother ruled the house, while my mother was subservient. It is still this way today in the small village of Akaovo, Greece, where my parents are from. I could see that my mother had no voice in our house. My father was important and so was Nikos. The males had penises, power, control, and love.

In one of my childhood dreams, I dreamt that my mother was sewing up my vagina with a sewing machine. Years later, an analyst would say that I once had a penis, but it was taken away! For a few years, I tried to urinate from a standing position to prove that I could do everything that Nikos could. Eventually, practicality forced me to accept my biological limitations.

There was, however, one special thing about being female. I was Daddy's little girl. He doted on me, and I basked in the glow of his attention. My father was a professor, but every Saturday he would spend the day with me. I was the apple of his eye. Unfortunately, as I approached puberty, my relationship with my father changed. As I started to sprout breasts, my father became uncomfortable expressing physical affection. He became remote and our Saturday outings came to an abrupt stop. The old angers smoldered inside me. I had no place to express the way I felt. This is when I started to keep a journal. I could write how I felt and be honest without getting punished.

I matured early, and at age thirteen, I looked about twenty. I decided to use my femininity as my new form of power. I dressed provocatively, wearing tight jeans that looked pasted on, and often went without a bra. I was a little girl in a woman's body and and I claimed my body as though it were a weapon that could help me attain power. There were always guys coming around, and I would purposely pick the least desirable young man. I had repeatedly been told that I was bad. So, I had nothing to lose—or so I thought.

When I got into high school, my insecurity and self-loathing had reached an all-time high. I was a first-class tease and hungry for power. The routine was simple and calculated. I would get some male's attention, and when I knew he was completely mine—Wham!—I dropped the guy like a hotcake. I had affair after affair, and started to collect notches on my belt for each man I seduced. I behaved exactly like a man; I used the opposite sex in a detached way, and after each conquest I rejected my prey. And then in my sophomore year, I met Ronnie, who was twenty-one and so ugly he was almost good-looking in an awful sort of way. For the first time, I was a love-sick puppy. Ronnie was every parent's nightmare. He was an ex-con who had served time for breaking-and-entering and dealing drugs; his mother ran a prostitution ring. At the beginning of our relationship, he proudly told me that he had knocked up his previous girlfriend so he wanted me on the pill. I complied. My father forbid me to ever see him, and my mother begged me to tell her the truth about my sexual activities. She warned me, "If you ever get pregnant, your father will disown you and he'll go to live in Vermont."

"Don't worry," I lied through my teeth, "I'm not having sex."

THE WORLD COMES CRASHING IN

I had the perfect ruse, or so I thought. Ronnie's best friend, Danny, was a clean-cut young man who would show up at my door and politely converse with my parents, who were delighted that I was dating a traditional preppie type. As soon as we left, I would sneak off to see Ronnie. This continued for almost a year, till Danny, who had his eye on me for himself, told my father the truth. I was forbidden to see Ronnie, but forbidden fruit is always sweeter. Threats didn't stop me.

When I was sixteen, my world came crashing in. I was pregnant. I had stopped taking birth control pills. I didn't tell my boyfriend. I had heard smoking was bad with birth control; at least this was my rationale. Years later, I realized that I did this by design. A part of me wanted to be pregnant. I'll never forget the moment that I heard the news. I was with my friends at a grocery store bagging groceries. The social worker called. "Your test was positive." You'd think I'd be devastated, but my feeling was pure joy. I had something—a secret that was hidden inside of me, and no one could take it away. I felt euphoric. The fantasy of having a baby was very satisfying. I had these wonderful symptoms. My breasts started to swell. I had morning sickness. Yes, even this was wonderful to me!

I still remember the exact words I wrote in my journal at the age of seventeen.

Journal Entry—February 14, 1988

I'm euphoric. I'm going to have a baby! I can't stop smiling. I'm so happy. Look what I've got growing inside me . . . a baby!

But within twenty-four hours a different reality set in: "They will never let me keep the baby. If I keep the baby, I will lose my family. As religious as Mommy is, she will still want me to have an abortion. How could they live with the shame? How could I?"

Journal Entry—February 17, 1988

I'm scared. I don't know what to do.

This was the last entry I made prior to the abortion. I knew I had to make the choice I did. There was no other choice. The fantasy was that I could marry Peter. Although he had offered, I knew it was a poor choice. My parents didn't like him—they tolerated Peter. He was twenty-one, and I was sixteen. He was not in my socio-economic class. Worse yet, he was verbally abusive, and was showing the beginnings of physical abuse. Nevertheless, I thought I was in love with him—I had been with him for one year before I did the procedure.

Since I was an only child, my mother was very involved with me. Curiously, my mother appeared to remain oblivious to my body changes and said nothing. On the day of the abortion I had to leave at 6:30 a.m. I told my parents that there was a family event at the police academy where my boyfriend worked. They seemed to buy this explanation. My boyfriend took me into Boston. You didn't even need parental permission. I went up a cobblestone path and saw a seedy-looking doctor smoking a cigarette. I was angry. I needed to give blood prior to the procedure, and I didn't want to give the nurse my arm. I was emotionally torn and asked for a priest. They said they would try to get one for me, but in the meantime, the procedure took place. I was not knocked out. They dilated my cervix. I still remember the sound of the vacuum. Afterward, I saw a bleached-blonde nurse taking away a jar filled with blood.

"Is that my baby?" I asked.

"No, it's just the blood," she replied. It would take more than two decades for me to write this poem:

The Cyclone

Darkness oozes a ferocious voice
insinuations of doom grease the
skyscape with your reckless habit
jeweled with envy you funnel
fury ensnarled threatening
to slash sturdy landscape
silence sounds a potent fear
coiled snakes ignite
couriers of sorrow
blurred bursts bruise
innocence leaving
vivid hues of
vacant souls
a murderous
spectacle
you
are!

After the procedure, I was very angry. I had wanted Mother to stop me; it was my fantasy that she would. My mother, who always hovered over me, made no mention of the fact that I was throwing up every morning. Nor did she seem to notice that my body had started to change. I wanted her to know what had happened. Afterwards, I bled for many days. I left a huge box of Kotex on my dresser. I never told my parents, but I am certain that my mother knew subconsciously. I left her many hints, which she never picked up.

When I returned home after the abortion, I told my mother that I had seen a neighbor on the way, and my mother said, "Oh, my Lord, she must have thought you were going in to have an abortion. (Gasp!) What would make me say a thing like that?!!"

Her conscious mind would not allow her to accept it. She was a devout Christian, an obedient wife and daughter, who was drowning in a subservient marriage. My mother was loving and generally wonderful, but sometimes emotionally distant. Her message, which she lived by, was: "Stuff it. Smile and the whole world smiles with you. Cry and you cry alone." My mother's inability to be there for me was a betrayal that I still carry with me.

Passive Tiger
The lilac blossoms
sour spilling
their hues
of grief unfinished.

Silent fragile
Mother watches
a passive tiger

does not reach
her paw to protect
her young.

Rather you are
frozen
in collusion.

The dampness of years
settles upon
shades of secrets.

You cannot offer comfort
choked
with betrayal.

Right after the procedure, I felt a sense of emptiness and sadness.[1] I wanted to forget it had ever happened. I had changed. I was no longer a child. I tried to go back to old friends I'd had before I got mixed up with a bad crowd. I still saw Peter. I tried to be happy. But my feelings about the abortion were never resolved.

I thought about seeing a priest and confessing, but in the Greek Orthodox tradition, confession is done face to face. My shame stopped me from doing that. However, in the Catholic confession, the priest does not see you. This was much easier. Two years later, at the age of eighteen, the priest listened to my confession and then said, "In life, what we must try to do is balance good with bad. Now, you should spend time working with disadvantaged children. Do twelve Hail Marys."

During my college years, I was a serious student. I had a pervasive sense of melancholy, but kept busy and was academically successful. I chose to become a special education teacher; it was a way of fulfilling the priest's directive.

NIGHT FISHING

In my senior year, I met Phil. At twenty-three, I had low self-esteem and thought I could only attract bad guys. Phil was different. He was the first man who was handsome and good. I felt a higher power was involved. He was goal-oriented, protective, loving and respectful. In short, he was all the things that I wanted in a man, but didn't think I was worthy of having.

We married. I became a special-education teacher. My work nurtured me, and at the same time was my penance. Phil worked in export/import trade and did a great deal of traveling overseas. My melancholy was triggered by feelings of abandonment when Phil was gone for long periods of time.

At such times, my grief would rise from the underworld of my restless dreams and almost always featured the ocean.

The waters are deep
swollen bursts seep
to the surface
slashing
I tread the unconscious
ocean overwhelmed
alone
fearful of the depths
that swallow me.

Some of my old behaviors started to resurface. In the school where I worked, I resented the male principal and male teachers who seemed to think their maleness guaranteed them privilege and power. I fell back again on my "cock-tease" routine. I dressed seductively and used my sexuality to bring them to their knees. All the while, I felt unworthy and angry. Dogged by a low level of depression, I entered psychoanalysis. It was an intense process; I went four times a week for an hour and a half over a five-year period.

The psychoanalysis was valuable, and helped me to attain insight, but it went only so far. It took many years for me to accept that God had forgiven me. It took many more years for me to forgive myself. I punished myself over and over with my own organic blend of biological martyrdom, in the form of ulcerative colitis, diagnosed by the age of twenty-three. My feelings were making their way through my body in a destructive way.

My ulcers continued to bleed sporadically, particularly at times when I felt deprived of my voice or unable to make a decision. One night I had a vivid dream that took place in an antiquated basement. The basement is my self-created hell, my purgatory.

In the Passion of my Bowels
On the outside
Nothing appears awry

A smile conceals

138

Though my silent tongue
Seeks release

In the passion of my bowels

Dreams explore

Endless rumbles
Of an antiquated
Basement
Secreting

Smoldering heat
From a furnace charred
With memory . . .

My work was a form of atonement, and an effort to be redeemed. I loved the children. They were thrown-away children that nobody wanted. But in my busy classroom, the children blossomed. We did arts and crafts, poetry, and music. It was a hands-on environment. In a vacant closet in the classroom, I kept "the jar." It was a half-filled receptacle well-known to the children because it held "tokens"—small rewards they received for good behavior. But this jar is a reminder . . . of another jar, another time.

The Jar

On a silent shelf
of a vacant closet
remains the jar.

Wide mouthed, reticent,
container of collections
comforting stones, childhood shells,
whispers of worn sea glass.

The same jar
turns bloodied
with the contents
of my womb.
An image held
twenty-two years
carelessly carried away
by a bleached nurse
exempt from truth.

Resolving the remnants
of my life,
I reach for the jar
half-filled receptacle
now containing colorful tokens of
my atonements.
Still the scream
of a vengeful cyclone
revives the horror
vibrating the truth throughout
my body sucking
what's mine from me.
The jar
is all
that's left.

My grief was repressed—it hid in a murky underground of dreams. During my waking life, I pasted a smile on my face. These damaged children became a part of me, but the work was draining. No wonder I once had a dream that I had multiple nipples. My analyst said that the children were sucking me dry. After fifteen years of exhausting work with autistic and emotionally troubled youngsters, I needed desperately to stop. I was torn by guilt about this decision. Curiously enough, the special children I taught inspired me to attempt writing. I tried to reach these troubled children with art, music, and hands-on projects. Surprisingly, I found that I could reach them through poetry. Poetry gave them a voice to express the anger and sadness. I thought perhaps it could do the same for me.

This poem was written about twenty-five years after the abortion. It was one of the first poems that I ever wrote.

My Regret

It was never enough that
  You
Forgave me
For the unmentionable sin

The words of the Catholic Priest
Echo my life—"Give back what you took."

Fifteen years
Of damaged children
Suckling
At my breasts
  Until
They drank me up

Their mouths opening and closing
Gasping, Wide-eyed
  Little fish
  Trying to breathe life

Because I could not speak
I held you in my gut
  All these years
  All these years

The inflammation
Tears of blood

A reminder
reminder
reminder . . .

In my dreams, I always saw an ocean or body of murky water. The feelings were disturbing. I would awaken from these dreams troubled. I started to write my dreams down. I was, in a sense, "night fishing," or waiting for a "catch"—an image that would help me to understand these murky feelings that clouded my dreams and left a sad, tacky residue during my waking hours. I turned more and more to writing and drawing.

My early experience of loss left me with a fear—a feeling that something I loved could be taken from me. I would wake up asking myself, "How can I be certain that God is not going to take something away?" I understood that this is the order of life; we cannot hold on to everything. In one of my dreams, I saw a beautiful rose in my garden. The rose dropped its petals without trying to hold on to them.

I am not a rose that accepts
The season of blooming.
I hold on to what I love
With tightly clenched fists
Riddled with fear
Of a force great enough to pry my hands free
One finger at a time.

How I envied that rose, so gracefully releasing its petals. When I was giving birth to my daughter, I didn't want her to be taken from me! I struggled with each contraction eagerly looking forward to her birth, but dreading the possibility of loss. Despite my fear, Phil and I were blessed with a beautiful little girl. Eventually I left teaching and became a full-time mother. The dreams and nightmares did not stop. The ocean was always present. But slowly they started to change.

Transformation
*Your waves of forgiveness
smooth the jagged edges
of glass memories
into muted glimmers
of green and rare
fragments*

*of blue
        hope I see*

in my daughter's eyes.

As I started to express my feelings more and more, my physical symptoms started to abate. When I wrote, I felt empowered. Writing was accessible twenty-four hours a day. Phil continued to be away much of the time, but I could always rely on my journal to be there. My mourning period had not yet come to an end. But writing was cathartic.

*Tears release
trinkets tainted
with bitter blood
until
        cleansing
                luscious language
                rains*

Slowly my body is healing. Something within me is changing. I feel lighter, as though the grief is no longer weighing me down. The nightmares rarely occur, and when they do, I convert my grief and fear to concrete art or poetry and am able to rebound quicker than before. I am now experiencing the world differently. I return to some of the same images that I had written about, but I see them with new eyes.

143

Transformation

Shark
Symbol of dread
Portending the most evil of happenings
Devouring destructive force
Leaking into my dreams
Fear

In a dream I stand
Within the vastness of the ocean

Lulled by its glossy rocking
I am caught unaware

The sharp black fin stuns
Cutting through water
Like the knife of a surgeon

Doom tarnishes my throat
I run against the current
My legs weighted down
With burdens of loss
Drained and parched I arrive at the shore

Years later
Inhaling healing salt air
My eyes are fixed on the great sea
That same black fin
Turns playful flips frolicking
Fear transforms into joy

Joy is something I have not felt for a very long time.
The grey veil of mourning
is now being lifted.

Joy, for too many years
You have been submerged
In a black sea
Crushed and confined
By walls of despair.

And now ancient walls
Eroding giving way
Icy layer beneath icy layer
Until shell after luminous shell
Peels to the innermost pearl.

This last poem signifies a turning point for me. I am finally able to let go of my guilt and regret. I feel blessed by my family. I am more vocal in my marriage; I have thrown away the shield of silence, passed down through the generations. I have begun to find my voice, and claim my own power.

The Jar II

The jar that once held my pain,
my regret, my flashback of horror,
has emptied its bloody contents.

The jar, no longer container
of childhood wishes
and colorful tokens of my atonements
nor, is this jar receptacle
of a dead specimen to grieve.

Wide mouth, no longer silent,
speaks of grief longstanding.
Lid, long held shut,
twisted tightly, gripping death,
has burst open with life.

Atonements become caterpillars
bulging with the joy of release
shedding their grief in layers.
Hanging still, now emerging
from winter's sleep as
mystifying monarchs.

Lid, there is no need for you now.
I will not hold on
I am letting go, letting go,
letting light burst forth
nourishing possibilities
nourishing promise
as pain transforms into beauty.

Butterfly, on the spirals of wind,
I release you.

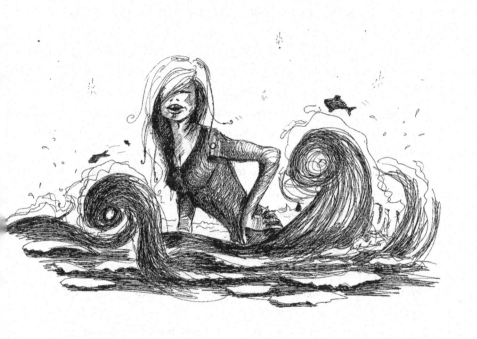

Nadia's childhood comes to a swift end with her pregnancy. It is a pregnancy that she herself has unconsciously engineered. Perhaps, as her analyst once said, it is an unconscious wish to have her father's child. Or perhaps it is an unconscious wish to give the nurturance she so desired for herself. In any case, Nadia's actions result in an abortion that must never be spoken about. What is repressed will eventually rise to the surface to be expressed.

Nadia's writing serves several purposes. Initially Nadia does not know the cause of her feelings of distress and nightmares. Therefore, she writes and paints for clarity and organization, as well as reflection and problem-solving. The paintings and writings become works of witness. Nadia uses her creative gifts in order to regulate her feelings of grief, anger and confusion. She seeks forgiveness and also writes for enhanced awareness. She yearns to connect to God, as well as the soul of her lost baby. Even when she feels that God has forgiven her, she still needs to forgive herself.

Unfinished business needs to be completed. Although abortion was the choice she made, her soul is tormented by her decision. "If I keep the baby, I will lose my family. . . . How could they live with the shame? How could I?" Integrating this event is complicated by the secrecy, guilt, and shame surrounding it.[2]

In a home of repression, members of a family collude with each other to make certain the secret does not see the light of day. For many years, the secret that Nadia carries is forced underground. It has been said that our memories are stored in our body, and the body will have its say. In her early twenties, Nadia begins to suffer from bleeding ulcers. Drops of blood, like tears, remind her of her spiritual debt. A low-grade depression motivates Nadia to enter psychoanalysis. She gains insight through the analysis, but still suffers from bleeding ulcers and is plagued by nightmares and restless dreams. In these dreams, the ocean (amniotic fluid? the feminine unconscious?) is a recurrent image that seems to hold the keys to Nadia's physical and mental well-being.

Some twenty-five years after the abortion, Nadia begins to write and draw the images of her dreams. Although she feels blessed by her marriage and the birth of a beautiful little girl, the nightmares continue. Her creativity is a driving force that empowers her and gives her a sense of mastery. With the freedom and safety of "poetic license," Nadia pushes beyond the confines of gender, culture, and religion to transcend her shame and guilt. Externalizing the trauma in words and images enables her to harness the healing power of her creative imagination.

Stanley Kunitz once said, "The imagination is a deep-sea diver that rakes the bottom of the poet's mind and dredges up sleeping images."[3] Only in the process of "night fishing"—through the sifting of watery dreams and the netting of important images and symbols—can Nadia retrieve the information she needs for her own unfinished healing. Each symbol and image is like a pearl, created out of psychic pain. Nadia works and reworks the elements of her trauma until she is able to integrate the disparate fragments into a whole.

Psychiatrist Dr. Jack Leedy once said that an ulcer is a poem struggling to be born,[4] and in Nadia's case this proves to be true. Only when the dream images are translated into written form is she able to come to terms with a decision made so long ago, a decision made without freedom, in fear, sorrow, and resignation. In creative freedom, her spiritual debt is finally laid to rest. After many deep sea expeditions, the joy that was submerged in the black sea for so many years is finally claimed—by the woman who went night fishing.

~ 8 ~

The Words That Built a Fortress
Richard Fireman

Self-image is created not only from how we see ourselves; it is created from how others see us and how we see them. We are reflecting mirrors for each other. The reflection mirrored in the mother's eyes plays a primary role in our concept of self. Even when we are adults, our parents still hold some of the threads from which our identity is sewn over time.

When Rich's mother is diagnosed with Alzheimer's,[1] she begins a rapid descent into severe dementia. Rich watches his mother deteriorate over a five-year period and it shakes the very foundation of his identity. At times, his mother looks at him with no recognition. Eventually she barely speaks. Words seem to have lost their meaning. The sharing of books and poetry, once a favorite pastime of mother and son, is no longer of value . . . or is it?

This is Rich's story.

INTRODUCTION

L ife doesn't develop according to formulas. Maybe that's one reason why at heart I'm a poet instead of a scientist, which I originally set out to be. I don't earn my living as a poet, either, of course; few do. Instead, I have tried my hand at different occupations, including working as a postman, a social worker, and a paralegal. Like many of my "lost" generation—the "baby-boomers"—I was at home more in academia than in the real world.

Early in college I had discovered a passion for writing poetry as well as reading it. I switched my major from physics to psychology to English literature, largely inspired and encouraged by a brilliant instructor of freshman English, the late Richard Leigh.

Morphing into adulthood in the crazy 1960s, I eventually got my B.A. I wrote hundreds of poems, many of which were philosophical or spiritual in nature, or simply attempts at trying to figure it all out. At any rate, poetry became a natural expression for me, and I turned to it in times of stress and to help express and process feelings, thoughts, relationship complications, frustrations, confusions . . . y'know: life.

My upbringing was unremarkable in most ways. My mother was, at best, difficult; very nervous, very overprotective, very insecure, very rigid in her ways.

I loved her immensely.

To paraphrase Walt Whitman: "Do I contradict myself? Very well, I contradict myself." My father was—like many of his generation—uncommunicative, and demonstrated little emotion. He was bright, but uneducated and downtrodden. He almost never spoke and was always tired, often falling asleep in front of the TV and waking up early to take the subway to work. He worked very hard, in New York's garment center, to provide us with a middle-class life-style in Brooklyn, and later in Queens, while my mother was primarily a homemaker. When Dad retired they moved to Florida.

In 1984 my father had a heart attack and passed away. Some time later, Mom remarried. Unfortunately, her second husband developed debilitating kidney disease. My mother somehow managed to "keep it together" for several years, until he eventually died eleven years later; that was the "straw that broke the camel's back." Within a few months, it seemed as though there was no longer an incentive for her will to maintain itself against her deterioration. Although we had noticed some memory loss the previous year, we hoped it was just the usual aging process. Instead, her confusion and memory loss greatly accelerated.

When I received a phone call from her accusing me of taking money from her and saying I wasn't her son, I knew something was very wrong. My wife and I went to Florida, had her evaluated medically [diagnosis: dementia], and began looking for an appropriate nursing home. After several months of mistreatment, we decided to bring her to a facility close to us, in New Jersey, and did so, visiting her every week for several hours and keeping close tabs on her condition.

THE CRISIS

When my mother's situation worsened and became critical, writing was a natural venue for me; the path was already established. Writing was comfortable and known; it was a ready tool and a steadfast, reliable companion. Along with my wife's invaluable support, my writing helped me keep it together.

In the first few poems I wrote to or about my mother, I was still coming to terms with the full brunt of the situation, with the loss of my mother's identity. Her loss of identity somehow affected my identity, as well as the relationship between us. I missed what my father and I had never really established; perhaps the pain of this vacuum served to strengthen the bond with my mother. Despite many differences and difficulties, from the beginning of my life, my mother was the one person who had understood me. She was my Rock of Gibraltar in a shifting world. It was a primary bond, always there for as long as I can remember.

I could not imagine my world without her. And yet I was faced with a mother who was not only losing her memory but her mind. A mother who imagined me to be conspiring against her, who saw shadowy figures in her lonely room, who thought both her husbands were still alive. And when medication was used to "fix" the misfiring neural circuitry of her brain, this was the result:

> Mouth eats
> in animal reflex
> Hands move
> do not grasp
> Lips speak
> words do not connect
> Eyes look
> but no longer see.

Ah, yes. We live in a time when we think we can fix everything, when we think it is no longer necessary to pray to the moon. A magic bullet for syphilis, a magic cocktail for dementia.

> I drink a glass of wine to my mother,
> to memory, I try to remember a time
> she knew who I was, knew she loved me.
> Today she said she did not know me,
> said she knew I was not her son.
> They said it was the medicine.

I was traumatized. Everything was stark, like a black-and-white Frankenstein movie I was watching but couldn't believe. I was told they were still adjusting her medication. But what I saw was that she was a robot—an animal with automatic reflexes but nothing that was her. No humanness. I felt starkly alone and at odds with a horrible universe that made no sense. I was devastated by her not knowing me. I wanted to believe that my mother's inability to recognize me was just due to the medicine, but my emotional intuition was whispering that this was just a rationalization to appease me.

Now, I asked myself, who was getting paranoid? I tried calming myself, I tried being rational in a *Twilight Zone*. I was trying to reconcile and accept it, but my intellect and emotions were at war with each other. I needed to communicate this, to assuage the pain.

How could I establish that I was her son? Now I was responsible for *her* knowing as well as my knowing, responsible for the validity of the relationship. Like a Tiffany egg I was trying to prevent from falling and shattering, I was responsible for the maintenance of this fragile person, this being who was and who was not my mother.

In systems theory and in relativity, when one part changes in a system, so does everything. My mother and I had formed a system. And now, like two planets revolving around one another, the decay of one was necessarily impacting the other.

> *There is a caliber of stone*
> *a moon of painted rain*
>
> *mind on cruise control*
> *when I'm with my mom*
>
> *different worlds*
> *like spaceships trying to dock*

Writing enabled me to take a step back; it was like being outside of myself looking in, as I was learning to adapt to my mother's changing circumstances. The writing enabled me to get a healthier perspective; the poetry served as my therapy. It allowed me to be conscious of the adjustment process, as recorded each step of the way.

From the nightmare period, early in the journey:

Visibility Zero
What are you thinking about, Mom?
No answer

154

was the answer.
The grooves were worn out
after so much turning,
they could not connect right
any more. Like a bolt turned
too tight too many times,
the thread was gone, lost,
like the TV picture gone to static,
radio to white noise, sunset
to the dark.

I was still struggling, still at war with what was going on, fighting reality. My mother was at peace—she had no choice—but I was not. The poetry was an attempt to make rational sense out of the meaningless static, like seeing imaginary shapes in the clouds. We create form out of chaos to feel more in control, even though we are not.

Shortly after my wife and I moved my mother to New Jersey, we arranged to have her few remaining possessions moved up here as well, and it was quite traumatic for me to unpack them, each bearing strong and concentrated memories.

Placement

My mother's life lies strewn in boxes.
They lie scattered around the room.

Painting I sent her returned to me,
Starry Night re-lit.

Ancient gold Chinese dragon spun by Russian nuns,
her inheritance passed on.

Shells we found when I was a child
washed up to a different shore.

155

Oriental scrolls, Russian spoon & egg,
jade Buddha, Solomon stone,
favorite books, old poems,
whale & teapot . . . the extents of a life
transported. The list is endless, the list
has ended.

Here I was trying to put my mother's life in boxes, sifting treasure from trash. The Van Gogh painting was a favorite of mine and hers. The ancient Gold Chinese dragon was from my mother's parents, one of the few things they'd managed to rescue from the pogroms against the Jews in the Ukraine. The shells we found on the Jersey shore when I was a child were finally returned to me, like a wave in the ocean returning.

Writing enabled me to apprehend these treasures as a whole rather than as separate, fragmented remnants of a life, which was my first—and upsetting—impression.

Recording these experiences helped me to integrate what was happening, to look at the larger picture. Setting it down on paper allowed it to germinate, giving it roots. At least this way my reality was substantiated; it seemed to make sense and I found a way to accept it.

Once the doctors adjusted the medicine, there was some improvement. There were "up" times when she seemed almost like her old self:

She gets the last applesauce.
"Why?" she asks.
"Because you deserve it."
She smiles
and a small world
> > *blooms.*

And then there were the "down" times:

New Worlds Need Names

This time it was all going well
but as we watched the TV
she said it's going too well,
something's going to happen.
At the end of the show I got ready to leave
and she asked me to take her home.

She was home. She didn't know
like she didn't know I came to see her each week
or what a galaxy was
or how to tear a tissue.
She couldn't understand how I knew she'd be there,
how I'd know what planet to point the ship at.

In the old days they were wise to make constellations
when they didn't know where they were heading,
to recognize what was too far away.

How do you tell someone that they have no home and that they never will? That they are helpless? That their identity is gone? This was not electronic identity theft. This was the real thing. I didn't—I couldn't—tell her, "You've lost your mind. You're in a nursing home." Usually I would just try to divert her attention. What else could I do? This was the way it was. Each such situation forced a mini-confrontation. I had to deal with it, but how? I found that, in order to emotionally deal with each episode, I had to write a poem afterwards to explain it to myself, to give it perspective and meaning.

I was creating a barrier with which to cope: with words, a medium with which I was comfortable. Words were the bridge still connecting me to my mother, even though they were no longer my mother's way of being in the world. For me, words were a necessary anchor to tether me to this world. I tried to erect a safety net of words against the fragments of harsh reality that threatened my mother. And myself.

Journey in Her Room

There are no more sentences
in my mother's life,
no more bridges for us to cross
the chasm. When she does speak
syllables tumble out like rocks, falling
this way and that.
She seems so lost, unconnected
in the world we make sense of,
homeless. I grab a book of Neruda
and cover her with his words
like a blanket.

It gives me more peace
than her.

Reading poems fights the noise
of the vacuum outside
and her silence.
Most I cannot read
because they speak of time or death or memory,
sickness and sadness, loss
loneliness or life,
all things too familiar to her
or too strange.

Sometimes fragments get through my net,
buzz at her like bad dreams.
When they get too close or too far away
she wheels herself to the wall.

I got in the habit of reading poems to my mother because I perceived that she liked me to do so. I don't know how much she comprehended, but it seemed to rekindle a pleasant mood that she partially re-experienced, re-creating the times when I had read poetry to her in the past, before she became sick. My mother had always encouraged my writing and interest in literature, and took solace and pleasure from that. If I could reproduce a fraction of that for her by reading poems—whether or not she was able to understand them—I did so. Still, I couldn't help but be aware of the inherent conflict and the disparity between the poems' content and my mother's lack of perception.

ADJUSTMENT

I am like Superman—my favorite childhood hero—trying to keep the relationship alive, but I'm racing against time. My mother is in her eighties and she's going to die. The ghost of death hovers in the air. Even in the frigid air of the Arctic, like the Northern Lights, I've been trying to protect myself against the loss of my mother, against the loss of my connection because, let's face it, losing hurts. The Fortress of Solitude was Superman's hideaway, and I created my own fortress to protect myself from the reality of the situation. My heroic efforts consisted of retreating into the mythos. I became the untouchable superhero, trying to be above it all. Metaphorically and psychologically, I inhabited an ice fortress, much like the one that Superman did. This was key to pretending—for years—that it wasn't hurting me. That I was safe. The poems helped me to confront myself in a bearable way. And then I suddenly realized I hadn't been using the word "love."

The Fortress of Solitude Is Where No One Can Find It

in twenty poems to my mother
I did not use the word love

frozen in the space of my fear
it hurts too much to connect

to feel the death separated only by time
the ghost that cannot be denied

159

This led me to focus on my own avoidance. It revealed the hurt I was trying to pretend didn't exist, the pain I was looking away from.

> "*How are you?*"
>> "*Not yet.*"

> *I try to hold my mother's hands*
> *but one is hiding in her sweater.*
> *I make a game of finding it*
> *like the game she must have played when I was a baby.*

> "*I love you.*"
>> "*I don't know where he is.*"

> *I talk to her, I talk to the nurse,*
> *I talk to the doctor, I talk to God,*
> *I talk to myself to try to understand.*

So Superman dared to make the big leap. Hey, he can fly. (It's about time!) This was the first poem in which I managed to bring myself to say "I love you." Perhaps I had realized the futility—or the pointlessness—of "protection." Or perhaps I was finally starting to accept that, indeed, no one has the answer. That perhaps there was no answer, just the seeking of one.

It took almost two years before I started to "have a handle" on circumstances rather than being at their mercy. I was starting to get used to this new life. Not only had I come to accept the way my mother was, but I had come to accept the way I must be: caring, but forced to remain at a distance. Words, however, had helped me to build a path to negotiate that distance, or at least make it bearable.

Last Request
The words leap into my mind unbidden
as though in compensation for the reality

she lacks.
Some things are not meant for sharing.
It is so hard to say goodbye,
take her last time away.
I feel I ought to give her more
and all I can give her now is time.

Random is as random does
but this was no accident.
She stared at what she did not see
and said two words: " life exit."

There is no science fiction like the present.

Once again we face the sun
& once again we shiver.

"Life exit"—there was a moment of weird prescience here, knowledge that comes out of nowhere. She seemed to be visualizing leaving life. This was one of a handful of poems which capture some of my mother's words as significant signposts, pointers to the fragmented world in which she resided. Every once in a while her synapses would connect, "click," sometimes in odd, incredibly meaningful ways. These expressions would capture the essence of what was going on for her, summed up in catch phrases that resounded with a frightening truth that was stranger than fiction. At such times she almost had a language of her own, and poetry was a means of translating that language to make it apprehensible in "our" terms, bringing it — and me—back down to earth.

When holidays would come, I was forced to confront the existential void in my life. I had lost one parent and was about to lose another. One Father's Day stands out in particular:

Celebration

It is Father's Day.
I am with my mother.
My father is gone and my mother is here.
My mother does not know where she is
or who I am. But we are together.

It is Father's Day.
I am with my wife.
I have come home from seeing my mother,
from seeing how far she has dropped.
My wife looks in my eyes, holds me. I cry.

It is Father's Day.
I am with my father.
He appears in the space between me and the stars
not there but imagined, not here but wished for.
He is silent as ever but says it's all right.

It is Father's Day.
I am with myself.
I am alone in the night and I walk in the woods,
stare at the sky, try to find stars.
There is nothing but clouds. I still try.

We delve into ourselves and find the past.
We delve into the past and find our selves.

I came home from the nursing home with "nothing but net"—not in a good way like a basketball player, but in the sense of a fisherman: an empty catch. Poetry enabled me to try to refill the net with something of value—to recharge my waning batteries, replenish my dwindling resources, and refuel my soul for my next trip.

There is so much to be said
and she cannot say much . . .

I don't want her to outlive me
I want to be there to hold her when she dies

I asked her if she's ready to go
and she said not yet, in a little while
and I don't know if she meant from the room or from life

she cannot say much but she did say
"this is the little center of time"

Another eerie quotation from my mother's lips, one that shook me in its simplicity and its appropriateness, while at the same time being very otherworldly, very much like something you'd find on the *Twilight Zone*. It's weird: she has three brain cells operating but comes up with philosophical profundities and then returns to silence drooling. You can't make this shit up.

ACCEPTANCE

Along the course of this journey with my mother, I experienced a shift of perspective, placing her in the greater context: she is one of the rest of us. I began to accept the universal significance of what was taking place. The next poem expands, as does my understanding, like a widening ripple in a pond, to include not only the subject but the poet, and even you, the reader.

I show her photos of the new kittens
but she does not know what they are.
She no longer has a problem with my taking her picture.
She used to be afraid of the image she'd project
but now there is no world to receive it:
neither gods to be offended
nor her.

Incapacity gives her freedom
at last.
And one day the old cat will be gone
and one day the kittens
and my mother
  and me
    and you.

None of us is exempt from fragility, illness, and death. As it is said, "There but for the grace of God go I." As I became more accepting of the situation, I was able to see my mother's plight in a more objective context. Thus, when another holiday arrived, and her condition had now deteriorated to a point where it would have been inappropriate for her to attend a family gathering, I was able to establish boundaries where they were needed, without being overly dramatic about it. My mother was surrounded by photographic images of the family she no longer recognized, and ironically, the family would no longer have been able to recognize the person she had become. It was kinder for everyone to hold onto their images of each other.

Now that the picture was clear—and accepted—it seemed to me I might be able to state things in a more succinct manner, and it occurred to me to try using the sublime form of the Japanese haiku [5-7-5 syllables] to force a concentration of the perception, and to create a snapshot of the total picture.

Mother Haiku
she is less each time
I visit the nursing home
each time it hurts more

The following matter-of-fact portrait, near the last days, somewhat fittingly occurred on Mother's Day, and this time I was reconciled to the situation.

Mother's Day at the Nursing Home

She sits in the hot sun in her three sweaters,
son by her side. Someone
takes their picture and leaves.
He opens a book and reads
while she stares into space
turning the pages of her life.

My wife returns with my mother
to where I am walking the dogs.
We all sit outside, eating the day
buttered like toast with the sun.

A few days later, my mother quietly passed away.

Now You Are Gone

There is no more railing at God
or blasting the blameless sun.
I have your permission and my own
to keep turning life's pages,
keep pace with the seasons.
The heart's pangs have their own rhythm:
no predicting when I will cry for the dead
or fall in love with the rain.

A baby's cry, a dog's wet nose,
ice water when the mouth is dry
can make me fall for the world once more,
put the covers on memory
and let it sleep its course,
and let me sing in the key of the wind.

The heart does not run according to timetables, after all. But it does run. It moves to nature's rhythm, like the earth around the sun, and to its own internal rhythm generated by the soul. In the warmth of my mother's love for me and mine for her, my world continued in its orbit; and in the wake of her loss, like the explosion of a distant galaxy, there yet remained an eternal reminder, like the constellations in the night sky.

In Greek mythology, Sisyphus seizes Death's pen so that Death cannot write the names of those about to die.[2] Similarly, Rich uses his pen in an effort to anchor himself to life and to sustain the connection between his mother and himself. He understands that Death looms ahead for his mother. Alzheimer's is a disease in which the death of the personality seems to precede the death of the body. Bereavement is complex and extremely painful as the personality we love dies but the body still lives.[3] It raises issues of our own mortality and the meaning of this life.

In Rich's ritual of daily writings, he records his feelings and perceptions. These writings serve as a reality check when Rich enters a dimension that feels like the Twilight Zone. Rich writes that he was "pretending—for years—that it's not hurting me. That I'm safe. The poems help me to confront myself in a bearable way." The poems shift time, space, and matter, giving the writer distance and safety. This distance helps Rich to clarify and affirm his perceptions so that he can deal with this situation in an objective and rational way. His purposes for writing are multiple: he writes for clarity and organization, reflection, witnessing, and integration.

Perhaps most important of all, he writes for a sense of security and protection. The writing provides a buffer for Rich; words form "a net" or "a barrier" against the harsh reality threatening his mother and himself. As Rich writes, "The poem . . . enabled me to focus on the hurt I was trying to pretend didn't exist, the pain I was looking away from." Writing creates a container for the painful material and, paradoxically, releases it at the same time, assisting Rich in the regulation of his emotions. Poetic license provides him with freedom and safety; words build a fortress around him.

Rich is very comfortable in the realm of writing, and returning to this medium gives him a sense of mastery despite the helplessness he feels in this situation. Like a miner in search of valuable ores, he continues to search for meaning as he delves—observing, recording, and reflecting on a situation that defies comprehension.

Rich evokes the archetype of Superman and the metaphor of the Fortress as a place of secret retreat, where he is untouchable. Rich's personal metaphors consistently suggest the other world that he has been forced to enter—e.g., "different worlds," "spaceships trying to dock," "Visibility Zero," "New Worlds Need Names," "Journey in Her Room." Rich is an explorer in an unfamiliar world that has a nightmarish quality "like a black and white Frankenstein movie."[4]

Words form the bridge that still connects him to his mother. As Rich says, "Words are a necessary anchor to this world." He continues to read poetry and stories to her in the late stages of the disease, even when he doubts she understands the words." I grab a book of Neruda / and cover her with his words / like a blanket. . . Reading poems fights the noise / of the vacuum outside / and her silence."

Sisyphus, of course, is not successful in cheating Death. It is said that he pushes a boulder to the top of a hill, and when it falls, he must start all over again.[5] Similarly, the process of caregiving in Alzheimer's is tedious, with little or no progress. It requires immense patience and emotional stamina.

Rich has two gifts that help him to cope. First of all, he has a large reserve of unconditional love for his mother. Secondly, his innate creativity is continually protecting him. He has a magic net—an intricate web of words (the magic of the poetic). He continues to work with his emotional inner life through his writing, strengthening his emotions through poetic exercises. Like a mountain climber, a net of words keeps him from falling into the abyss of loss and depression, and at the same time, tethers him to the world he still loves. He is able to remain strong throughout this difficult period of time because he has excellent resources; he has the support of his wife, good friends, and a multiplicity of words—the words that built a fortress.

167

~ 9 ~

The Woman Who Changed a Triangle into a Circle

Barbara Bethea

Every survivor has passed through one or more doors, where a new life has opened. Barbara stands in her new life every day, amazed and grateful. But the memories of another existence—a place of violence and terror—is just behind the door. At times, a sound or smell wafts through the door, reminders of the destructive life left behind. It is a life she has never forgotten. Barbara is a survivor of domestic violence. According to Domestic Violence Statistics in New York City, police responded to 229,354 domestic violence incidents in New York City in 2007; this averages to over 600 incidents per day.[1]

This is Barbara's story.

INTRODUCTION

I was born into a void. There was nothing for me to hold onto after I slid through the birth canal. I was my mother's fifteenth child. My natural mother was thirty-nine years old when she had me. She had married a man named James when she was sixteen years old. After having seven children with her husband, she left him. She met a man named Moses, who was married with children, and had eight children with him. I am the last child of this union. They had a very volatile relationship, which included alcohol, drugs, sex, and physical abuse. My mother left this relationship while she was pregnant with me. She had emotional problems and was not financially equipped to take care of her children. Most of us ended up in the foster care system.

At the age of four months, I was given to my foster parents. I grew up in a relatively functional home: no alcoholism, gambling, or irresponsible behavior patterns. My mother was a homemaker and my father worked for the U.S. Postal Service until retirement. My foster parents took in several other children, but there were four of us who stayed permanently. I had two other sisters and one brother. Visits to my biological mom gave me a bird's eye view of my mother's world of confusion and disorder, and I returned from these visits relieved and glad to have a foster family.

My foster mom was a powerful personality who did not allow dissension and believed in physical discipline. Everything and everyone belonged to Mom, and early on I went seeking my own true self. Perhaps that is how I first found my pen; it was a way I could express my thoughts without punishment. At the age of seven, I started writing poems and short stories, as part of school assignments and reflections of poems by Robert Frost, Christina Rosetti, and others. I wrote about the seasons and general matters. Towards pubescence, my writing began to focus on my own identity crisis, Black pride, and self-esteem issues.

THE TEEN YEARS

As I became a teenager, two aspects of me evolved. One aspect was the popular life of the party girl. It was important for me to be attractive, well dressed, and popular—a girl who was the life of the party. The other aspect was a superhero, a rescuer who saved the day. This supergirl was not necessarily loved, but I was needed. This meant I was important to others; I could not be excised or thrown away.

I had a strong desire to be a part of the unruly crowd, you know, people who were drinking, fast-talkers, loud and disruptive. Perhaps I just wanted to feel closer to the people I came from. Or perhaps these were personality traits imparted through the womb, passed on through my parental gene pool.

Well, I would get my chance to be a part of the unruly crowd, all right. I met Lafayette at a neighborhood party one week before my seventeenth birthday. Months later, I would find out he had just gotten out of jail that week. Here I was the lonely, horny, depressed, attention-starved teenager looking for love in all the wrong places. He just seemed so right. How could I say, "No"? I was too afraid and too lonely. I had someone to call my own and now I needed to keep him.

> *More than the smiles he seems to wear*
> *Or the style of his hair*
> *You need to know the heart inside*
> *The thoughts that flow within his mind.*

As time went by, I discovered that I had hit the jackpot. Not only was he into street life, but he was also an intravenous drug user. Wow! I made it to the big time. He became the first rescue mission in my life. I was going to help this person that no one else seemed to understand better than I could. He began to ask for and take money from me. When I didn't have it, he became abusive and slapped or threatened me with other women. I still couldn't say, "No." I was in way over my head. I began smoking a little reefer but that was as far as I went. I wasn't that curious.

> *More than the secrets he reveals*
> *More than the way he makes you feel*
> *You need to know what makes it real*
> *What makes the matter if it isn't real?*

THE SEARCH FOR LOVE

I graduated in June of the following year, and he violated parole and ended up back in jail. Saved by the bailiff? I kept moving forward in my life, but the pattern of dating remained the same. These were the best lovers I'd ever encountered, and I could play rescuer and save them from their plight with my all-encompassing love. See, I had enough love for the two of us. You didn't need to reciprocate; just act "as if" you loved me and I was comfortable. Say the right words, make the right moves, and give me all the sex I needed. Thank you. Goodnight. Next! What's love got to do with this any way? Thank you, Tina. I never felt I deserved love from a man or deserved anything. My mother gave me away shortly after birth. How worthy could I be? That's right—me, tall, black, ugly foster child.

I was leading a lifestyle filled with men, smoke, and wine. I desperately wanted to fill the void. I wanted to prove myself all-loving and indispensable. I was hungry for love, and that hunger dictated my actions. What did I want? Just to fill the hole in my heart.

> *Years from now beyond the laugh*
> *When passions cease and time has past*
> *You need to know where were you when*
> *The stranger entered and came within*

TRAPPED

After eight years of separation from Lafayette, I saw his aunt on the train one day. I gave her my contact information. She relayed the message. Perhaps a year later we reunited. He had lived in the south for most of those years and had left the drugs alone, but not the alcohol. I had had a daughter by another abusive partner. My daughter and I were living in Brooklyn in our own apartment. One day, Lafayette flew in to New York and began to live with us. I wasn't ready for this transition but, once again, I couldn't say,

"No." At first things were calm, but then the change took place. He began to come home later and later or not at all. When he did come in he was angry and began to yell and curse at me, followed with a physical assault. He became an addicted, womanizing, abusive bastard again.

> He used to beat me day and night
> As if I didn't matter,
> It robbed me of my self-esteem,
> It left my nerves a tatter.

My daughter suffered by his hands, as well. He plucked her in the head, and at times threw things at her. She bore witness to some of the beatings her mother took. I felt powerless, shamed, and guilt-ridden during this time. I met neighbors who remarked, "I was sure that you were killed last night. Are you all right?" Still others, mainly women, sneered with a sly grin, feeling superior over me because they were sleeping with him. The shame and guilt were overpowered with this false sense that, if I could just hang in there, things would be better one day. A false sense of pride also overtook me because I didn't want to appear a loser. I had always carried myself in a dignified fashion and had expressed such high ideals. How could this happen to me? If I gave up, then I was truly weak.

> I was a broken spirit,
> A shatter from within . . .

I stopped writing in my journal once violence took over my life. I was no longer a free woman, no longer free to explore my thoughts or feelings. I was growing smaller and smaller with each beating. I had no words. I was just trying to stay alive.

There was the dreaded anticipation that would overwhelm me sometimes as I listened to the key in the lock or footsteps coming towards the door. There were the nights that he would come home, beat me out of a sound sleep, and make me stay awake listening to his ramblings. Days and nights of surreal events that blended into one another. Once again, I couldn't say no. The sex was good, and the fear was overwhelming but maybe, just maybe, he might change his ways. If I didn't see this through, someone else would gain. Therefore, I stayed, cried, and lied to others and myself.

My warmth declared
A hot-zone of anger from you
Followed by the pursuit
Of sexual gratification
As if my wounds rewarded
You pleasure
Shaking and quaking, like vomit
Your sick desire
enfolded in me.

In a burst of hopefulness, I painted the hallway entrance a chocolate brown and orange. This was a reflection of my innermost soul. No one could save me from my plight but me and I knew it.

GETTING OUT

One day, I decided this was it, and I was prepared to put him out and end it once and for all. I found out I was pregnant and my heart sank. I tried to seek an alternative but could not go through the process. I confronted him with the fact that in spite of the pregnancy, I would make it with or without him. I was four and one-half months pregnant, and he still was hitting me. Finally, he left one evening and did not return until I was in my eighth month. I was devastated because I now had to face my pregnancy and the reality of my situation alone. I continued to care for my daughter, my unborn child, and myself, at first through tears, shame, and doubt, but eventually I gained confidence. I continued working until two weeks before my son was born.

I was twenty-nine years old when I had my son. His father took me to the hospital that morning and returned two days later to pick me up only after some coaching from my family. I came home, perhaps in postpartum depression, and began to sit in the dark and let my son cry in his crib. His sister became his caregiver and provided comfort to him when I refused. His father only came home sometimes, and when he did it was a nightmare. When my son was four and one-half months old, I ran off to Baltimore with my children to my sister's home. After two months, I came back to him in New York and returned to work. We would remain together for a few months more and then break up for good. Each time things went from bad to worse. I ran out of excuses in my head and finally was able to step away from this relationship.

Then Jesus took me by my hand
Became my dearest friend.

I used to live with misery,
Engulfed by fear inside.
There was no sanctuary,
No place to run and hide.

We were having sex one day, and as he thrust into me, I thought about the methodical rhythm of his body and began to snicker, which turned into laughing in his face. This touched his manhood and became a turning point, in which we realized I was no longer under his influence and was gaining a sense of self and pride.

RECOVERY

I had begun to attend church during this time and was replacing the powerlessness with Holy Ghost power. I heard that Jesus Christ was the hope of glory in a person. Not far away on a hill or in outer space but in one and that a person could be strengthened from within. The repetition of this message of hope gave me hope. The fellowship and communion of others along with the inner and outer glow of love and peace wove itself around my heart and mind. I was set free from the spirit of bondage and took hold of the spirit of peace, power, and love.

> *But then a door was opened,*
> *A light that shone within,*
> *For Jesus took me by my hand,*
> *Became my dearest friend.*

> *I never thought my hurts would heal,*
> *I never thought I'd love again,*
> *I felt I had abandoned me*
> *That life was at an end.*

Eventually, I would join a women's group at church. Their experiences were varied and I felt comforted in knowing that I was not the only one who had suffered a traumatic experience in life. Some of these women had moved beyond the events of pain in their lives, which helped bolster my confidence levels. They were enjoying new relationships through God, themselves, and others. If God could forgive them and allow them to be free from guilt and shame, I learned that I could be blessed the same way. I began visiting them in their homes, going on retreats. My soul had been beaten into silence for years, but now a light glimmered for me. I started writing again, re-discovering my voice. I expressed myself in spiritual poetry. Some of these writings were performed in the church; others became a part of my healing process, as reflected in poetry.

> *But now I walk with confidence,*
> *With love, with courage, with pride,*
> *For Jesus came and washed away,*
> *Each hurt, each hate, inside.*

175

Despite my inner change and newfound strength, I had not cut my ties with Lafayette completely. The final episode occurred one day when new windows were being installed in the apartment. Large sheets of glass were placed around the apartment, and he became provoked by something said or done and began to attack me. Right there, right in front of the men installing these windows! Like it was a brotherhood or something. At one point, I was knocked to the floor, and my head barely missed going through the sheet of glass. It was a miracle. One of the men shouted out, "Yo, man, be careful of the glass, man." Not, "Stop hitting that woman like that!" or, "Why are you beating her like that?" Instead, "Be careful of the glass." Perhaps had there been some sort of accountability for his actions by the community and others, he may have considered stopping this behavior. I may have felt supported as well, but that never occurred.

So, he snatched me up and pushed me in the bathroom to finish what he'd started. He made a comment about hoping that my mother dropped dead. At the time, both of my mothers were still alive. I became enraged. That rocked me to the core of my soul, and I stood up to him and shouted in his face, "Which one of my mothers do you want dead?"

Something in my eyes told him that I was no longer afraid and would stand up for myself. He began to search behind his back for the doorknob to the bathroom. We were in a tight space, and it was getting tighter by the minute with the hate and anger I felt towards him. He finally got out of the bathroom and continued walking out of the front door, never to return. That was the last time we lived together. He married another woman about a year later. Eleven years later, he died of AIDS.

> In the silence, I hear the echoes
> Of screams and cries from
> My yesterdays
> That with each passing blow
> The thunderous fall of
> Furniture falling around my
> Head

Barely missing me,
Almost dying.
Immediately come the thoughts
Of safety
That comforts me
Heavenly spirit of Grace and Mercy,
That ordered angels to protect me,
I thank you.
When I wake
I no longer cringe and cower
In this inner darkness.
Where fists flew
Like shattering shards into
My open face, slaps of dominion . . .
You, a funnel of terrorized
Love notes.
Choiceless words and moments
That I never want to live through
Again
Whatever the path that led me to you
Let it be burned and blotted
From returning
When I waltz past these memories
They are the shadows of my mind's eyes
Music that stole the joy of rhythm
Words that robbed the passion of poems
Thoughts that drip the blood, pain, and fears
Of survivors that talk and
Those who can't,
Those now who walk into the sun
Did it ever occur to you
That my spirit is voice and
My tears are the rivers that washed

My freedom whole?
Did you realize that you would become
A vapor
Disappearing forever
To the nowhere from whence you came?

I was thirty-two years old, starting over, yet empowered with the will to win. I did not end up a loser. If anything, I gained a life I had not known how to live, along with the ability to say, "No." With this newfound freedom, my life and my children's lives began to soar. I began a new path towards healing and recovery that yielded many fruitful directions. There would still be personal demons to conquer and other bridges to cross, but the cycle of physical abuse was destroyed within me.

Facing myself would take on new meanings. Women's circles, spirituality, journaling, talking, and sharing my feelings with others through poetry and essays, helped me to overcome my darker side, by the grace of God. I amaze myself at times when I think of all of the obstacles I have overcome in my life and the personal growth and strides I have made to reclaim my personal freedom and peace of mind.

I've known the voice of silence
I've known the tortured years
When I had lived through violence
And lived through tears of fears.

I've known the sleeplessness of nights
Where deep inside I hid
The overwhelming sights
And memories of things I did.

The sounds of children crying
Avoidance in their eyes
Silhouettes of dying,
Days and nights of bitter lies.

I've known the voice of triumph
The sound of letting go
The many arms of comfort
The power to say no.

I sing the survivor's song
Of life over the raging tide
That washes over every wrong
And keeps me safe inside.

Today, my children and I are all on a path of discovery and recovery. We laugh, cry, and share our pains together as a family. When finally I was able to acknowledge my own beauty and worth, I attracted a wonderful and purposeful man in my life. My husband, Tony, esteems and cherishes me daily. We have opened our home to others in need, and we share a faith-based lifestyle. My self-worth is no longer mitigated by what someone else feels or thinks about me. I have become my own best friend. I believe the poet Mary Oliver spoke the truth when she said, "The only life you can save is your own."

I no longer live in pain, although the painful memories will always be there. Every survivor makes a choice. Some victims don't know how to separate themselves from the trauma. They wear the trauma like a cloak for life, and it chokes them. I have chosen a different path. I exhale the trauma every day.

I inhale Life.

Being separated from one's birth mother exerts a profound influence on one's life.[2] In Barbara's words, " I slipped through the birth canal and had nothing to hold onto." From the time she can read, books are what Barbara holds onto. Words are a source of nourishment, intellectually and emotionally. Most importantly, words are a way for Barbara to explore her identity and discover her own voice. She writes originally for the purposes of self-affirmation and nurturance.

The foster home is a full, hectic home with many other foster children. Barbara's voice often clamors for attention. It is a strict home and if rules are broken, or improper words are spoken, there are dire consequences. Her journal becomes a safe haven where Barbara can claim her own emotional space without interference or judgment from the family. When writing, Barbara exercises the five freedoms that Virginia Satir wrote about.[3] It gives her the space to know what she knows, feel what she feels, believe what she believes, experience what she experiences, and want what she wants without any repercussions. In a world where things seem out of her control, Barbara takes pride in her reading and writing.

As Barbara becomes a teenager, she describes how two aspects of herself evolve. Although one persona is a party girl, the other is a rescuer. "This meant I was important to others; I could not be excised or thrown away." Unfortunately, when she takes on the role of rescuer, Barbara enters a dangerous triangle. Dr. Stephen Karpman, a physician psychiatrist, specifies that there are three roles in The Drama Triangle: the persecutor, the rescuer, and the victim.[4] At any point in time, any of these three roles may switch, creating drama, and in this case, trauma. In fact, Karpman's Drama Triangle is a theoretical construct that accurately reflects Barbara's situation. Barbara enters her relationship as a "rescuer," and then becomes Lafayette's victim. Had she stayed in a violent relationship and fought back physically, she would have become a perpetrator. Drama games generate excitement, but undermine accountability, personal power, and rational thinking.

Domestic violence is a dance of power and helplessness, an intense blame game in which all freedoms of the victim are denied. During this period of violence, there is no writing because Barbara's voice, along with the freedom to say what she thinks and feels, has been obliterated. The only way to stop being a victim is to step clear of the triangle to a place that is free of all three roles. Although some people spend their lives within this power triangle, Barbara extricates herself from the triangle through her faith in God and the help of a supportive sisterhood of church friends.

When Barbara begins to heal, she reclaims her voice and she is able to write again. Her writing then serves a vital function; it is a witness to the trauma. Barbara tells her story through narrative poetry, in a style reminiscent of singing the blues. The return to the past becomes possible through the shifting of time, space, and matter, and Barbara writes to process and integrate traumatic memories.

With domestic violence in the past, Barbara writes to access a greater consciousness. Ultimately she connects to a spiritual power that is greater than herself. The reclaiming of voice—through writing, singing, and prayer—is crucial to her recovery. In poetry, hymn, and song, there is one consistent nurturing medium through which she connects to mother, father, community, and God—words. Whether spoken or written, words are the connectors that carry the nourishment like an umbilical cord connecting to mother, father, community, God, and most importantly herself.

From a Freudian perspective, Barbara has found her father in the Great Almighty and her mother in the circle of women who accept her. Barbara's feat is no less than a geometric wonder—somehow she has managed to transform a triangle of victimhood and helplessness into a circle of acceptance and empowerment.

~ 10 ~

The Woman Who Built a Labyrinth with Words
Susan Riback

Although we often believe our personal life story is sacrosanct and mostly under our control, there are times when culture, legal systems, and community have the power to fragment personal narratives. Sometimes the public tale overtakes the private one. Or a family member is in crisis and their disrupted storyline completely alters our own.

Susan was a nurse who married a handsome doctor and created a beautiful home in the suburbs where they were raising their two daughters. In 2003, Susan's husband, a pediatric neurologist, was accused of molesting his young patients and was imprisoned. Overnight, the American dream turned into a nightmare.

Isaac Bashevis Singer once said, "Life is God's novel, so let him write it!" Does Susan have the power to revise and edit the story of her life or is the story dictated from another source?

This is Susan's story.

INTRODUCTION

I t is now six journals and three years since the night my husband was questioned in the parking lot outside his office. The image of Phillip sobbing in my arms on the day he is released on bail is etched in my memory. I continue to replay various scenes in my mind. His account of the nightmare that comes in broken words: orange jumpsuit, shackles, eating spaghetti with a plastic spoon. In an envelope his personal belongings, his wallet and wedding ring, which he hasn't taken off for fifteen years. On his face is a hurt that he can find no words for; that is where I begin, looking for the words for a condemned man.

Yesterday Philip was a devoted pediatric neurologist—a healer, a scientist, known to diagnose rare diseases that other neurologists missed. He was highly respected and all the doctors in the area sent their own children to him.

Almost overnight, he lost everything. The news and the sensationalized media coverage escalated quickly. In a very short time, Phillip's life resembled that of Job in the Bible. He encountered loss after loss: his name, his career, his integrity, his home, and watching his children growing up.[1]

Losses like this are only tolerable with a journal in hand. There is so little control or power I have right now to change the situation. However, in my writings, the flow of life experiences is fluid, moving between the past, the present, and the future, which is where our hope lies.

Living through a traumatic story and carrying it inside me, I feel like a child who has a secret. Honestly, sometimes I just want to run up to a stranger and blurt, "My husband has been falsely accused and convicted of a crime he never committed and lives in a maximum security prison." (All in one breath!)

THE EARLY YEARS

I was never any good at keeping secrets. I was the youngest of four, and it was my role in the family to help keep the peace and harmony. I was born during the darkest days of winter, the size of a small baby chick. I was left to finish my growing in an incubator. I suppose I was an early survivor and such was the joy when I came home from the hospital that I was named "Susan Joy." Like a self-fulfilling prophecy, I enjoyed making others happy. Years later, it would be one of the reasons for going to nursing school. As a highly sensitive, over-empathetic child, I was told I was too "emotional" and was laughed at for being so tearful. I felt a deep loneliness that resulted from feeling misunderstood. It seemed like everyone was too busy to listen to my thoughts and feelings. My sisters, being much older than I, were busy with sports or dating. My brother, three years older than I, although a great friend, had his own adolescent struggles with mom and dad. It wasn't until I was in high school that I began writing in a journal. In these journals, I listened to myself and began to learn how to take care of my own needs. In these journals I could feel everything around me. I had the safety of a lined page in a blank book. I had time to re-read myself until I found the understanding that I wanted from others. More than twenty-five years later, these pages continue to keep me on course.

ACCUSED

It is the most difficult evening I have ever had to live through. Phillip calls to tell me he wasn't able to pick up our daughter because he is being taken to the local police station and is under arrest! He explains that some disgruntled patients have accused him of something, but he has no idea what he is being accused of. Meanwhile, on the evening news, the police chief stood in front of the camera and told the community that my husband was guilty of inappropriately touching two of his patients. They posted my husband's mug shot on the news and the phone number of the police station, alerting the community to call this number if they knew anything.

Phillip spent the night in the county jail. I was in shock. I was able to break through the numbness with these words:

Journal Entry—November 6, 2002, 6 a.m.

False Arrest
I hope you don't have one of those long sleepless nights
when the sun comes slowly and the rain comes
to deepen the sadness
not your name in the morning news
not you unable to watch the sun rise
surreal sun
unreal sun
after one of those nights
changes your life
forever.

I struggled that night. As if I were a wound up toy, I went through the motions of cutting the pomegranate, laying out pajamas, brushing teeth, and tucking in. I could feel the sky opening up and lightning striking us. I could feel the past, the present, and the future colliding in a matter of moments. I could feel the current of something larger than our small life rushing in and rising to overtake us.

Journal Entry—November 7, 2002

Last Night
Julia did the only thing an eight-year-old can do
in the presence of a pomegranate
even if her father was not coming home
even if the world was quickly drying up
to her it was a handful of hope
all sanguine and spilling into jewels
tasting juicy

I could not eat one seed
God was hiding in that pomegranate.

I busied myself in a frenzy of housecleaning. There was something calming about sorting the laundry and going through the ordinary routines of housekeeping.

After the Fact

Oh, it's bad all right
I line up all the shoes in the house
start a new load of laundry
sort darks from lights
wipe down counters

Only six in the morning
my God, I am no longer a child
I do not cry
I curse the world . . .
and straighten up the magazines.

During the next ten months, I sort out feelings like laundry. I make piles of poems. Some of them are prayers, others are letters, and many are descriptions of my daily struggles. I don't want to forget what I do not understand. I am collecting the feelings. Phillip is collecting newspaper articles. The lawyers are collecting evidence. Everything is so confusing. Worst of all, life goes on. The president is waging war in Iraq, our teenage daughter is the talk of the school for kissing a boy who belonged to her best friend, and our eight-year-old is falling for the star of the middle school play, the ugly duckling turning into a swan.

Everything "normal" is gone. I am in a heightened state racing against the forces of evil. Nothing matters except the swirling stories that are being amplified by the passing of months and in the interviews by the police, one newspaper after another. We experience a growing sense of powerlessness and disbelief that our life is becoming bigger than ourselves. We are not living this story; it is as if a story is living us. A drama beyond imagination is taking our identity, and challenging us to dig deeper for some part of us that no one can ever take away.

Journal Entry—November 8, 2002

> *Imagine one morning*
> *your face on every TV screen*
> *the name you were last called by*
> *coming from every car*
> *imagine a story of lies*
> *in place of your life.*

Not everyone believed the press. For the friends who came to our house with food and wine and hugs, for the friends who wrote letters and sent cards and brought over dinner, I wrote this poem. To this day, a friend tells me she still has the poem hanging on her refrigerator.

For Our Friends
> *who opened their arms to catch our fall*
> *as we had no choice*
> *but to jump from the roof*
> *of our burning hearts*
>
> *How else could we have landed*
> *without breaking,*
>
> *without shattering*
> *into a million*
> *unmendable pieces?*

There is no longer disbelief as there once was. In the beginning I wrote desperately to give voice to a situation that left us speechless. I didn't think we would be asked to remain silent, but we were told to save our thoughts for the trial. The only place for me to have a voice was through writing. I wrote "What We Need" so I could mail it to neighbors and friends; I wanted our community to understand our suffering and not believe everything they read in the paper. There was no defense for my husband that could withstand the power of black-and-white newsprint, and the accusations on prime time news.

What We Need

Need you to tell the world—Don't listen!
reporters banging on our door
strangers reading the headlines
from one sided stories

When they ask "Don't you know them?"
tell them before they take down our hearts
our buoyant hope

Need you to tell the world
to hold our hands in a chain of trust
you who know our sweet spun children
Tell them
of the delicate web that connects us
here where our children learned to speak
here where our name was fondly recognized

Need you to tell the world
lies are brewing over us
like a dark storm

We need you
to stand watch with us
and if the roof of our dreams
should be destroyed
please shelter us from the rain.

When Phillip is out on bail, his ex-partner, Chris, and his wife, Betsy, invite us to stay the weekend at their home on Martha's Vineyard.

Just the two of us, we walk to the lighthouse, along the dunes, beside the wind-shaped junipers, along the seagulls' footprints. We are warmed by the low sun. I want to forget everything, our whole life coming to this: sautéed onions, translucent and aromatic, two glasses of Cotes-du-Rhone, red French wine, candles dancing in the living room. What are we to toast to?

Journal Entry—December 30, 2002

Will this be the last time we follow the evening's light to its end,
driving down the long twisting road to Lambert's Cove?
Will this be the last time we walk over sandy dunes,
wide yawning beaches, blue sky,
emerald ocean startling green?
Will this be the last time we are alone,
being our best for each other?
Cooking our meals together
reading by the fire
singing old songs?
We hold on to the lonely buoy bell
ocean washing over the shore.
We must come back to this private road
this off season,
clam chowder and rolls
ferry going out, coming in,
leave us here forever.

In the gift shop at the Red Lion Inn in Stockbridge, Massachusetts, we come upon a book of love letters written throughout time. Phillip and I open spontaneously to a letter written one hundred years ago by Alfred Dreyfus to his wife while he was incarcerated at Devil's Island for a crime of treason he did not commit! In one letter Alfred writes, "We were so happy! All of life smiled upon us. Do you remember when I said we could envy nobody anything? Position, fortune, mutual love, adorable children . . . In a word, we had everything."

We were stunned by these words that could have been spoken from our mouths. Alfred, much like Phillip, referred to an "awful unexpected thunderbolt, so incredible, indeed that even now I sometimes think that I am the victim of a horrible nightmare." With these letters in our hands, we were warned of a possible future where we too might end up separated and writing such letters.

Journal Entry—January 1, 2003

> Thus begins a new year. January is cold and dark, but darker yet is this side of humanity that we are seeing for the first time. False rumors, cruel strangers, radio shows feeding the frenzy of media attention. The fictitious tales continue to grow.

An Acrostic for Darkness
Deeper than a casual conversation
A yearning to understand what is
Real in a world that is not
Kind, you will find me
Nearly laughing with the currents of
Electricity.
Startling, if your eyes have not become dark adapted.
So, welcome both the darkness and the light.

Hanging on for dear life, we thank God for each other, our home, our humor, and our steadfast hearts. Yet this hand of fate is playing us, taking away what we knew held us safe and secure. I cannot go back to the places I have been—not to exercise class, not to a house of worship, not to any public place. Phillip surrenders his medical license, packs up his office, his black leather doctor's bag gathering dust in the corner of the living room.

Journal Entry—February 2, 2004

> *With their huffing-and-puffing*
> *blow-your-house down*
> *and the smoldering of our hearts*
> *leaving us speechless,*
> *I wait for the words*
> *"It's safe now,*
> *Okay to come out."*

Only three weeks away from the trial, I wrote the following journal entry, hoping to find words that would give me comfort and courage. I do not take comfort easily from others. Perhaps it is my own sense of pride. I will offer a poem or speak from a deep place only after I have seen and read these private thoughts first.

Courage

What fear is this that swirls inside our stomachs?
My own? Phillip's? The girls'?
I carry the bundle of fears like women in Africa
Baskets of fear balanced on my head

Fear folded into sundried sheets
Still warm
Fear washed clean in the river
Fear blown into the wind by a soft breeze
Fear returning to the sky.

What fear is this that takes hold of our life?
Move it into open fields
Let the hungry falcon come to take it
From our home.

SENTENCED

After ten months of waiting for it to become apparent that this whole thing is a mistake, it becomes clear that not only will that never happen, but instead more children are being interviewed as possible victims! The police are building a case against Phillip, and one police officer is heard saying, "No matter what, we will get him on something."

With great fear, my husband hears of the grand jury's decision and is taken before the judge to be indicted. He pleads, "Not guilty." The press is vicious and news cameras follow too closely for him to walk down the court halls. He leads one cameraman into a corner and escapes a microphone thrown in his face. We do not watch the evening news.

Offering

Neighbors are whispering
"He's that man in the paper . . ."

"the prominent neurologist . . ."
"those poor boys . . ."
It's like the old village
children throw stones
people in the streets turn silent
when we walk by.
Oh the mind of the masses
the medieval gallows set
crowds shouting
"Admit the crime!"
They want to put my husband away
hang him
burn him
destroy his life.

We don't want to be
a part of this world.

I believe in Phillip. I believe in his innocence. He does not belong in prison! Yes, he used poor judgment—wrestling on the floor in play—but I know there was never any intention to sexually touch his patients. Ironically, Phillip's high moral character was one of the reasons I fell in love with him.

IMPRISONMENT

I can't get my arms around the prison thing. Even as I walk toward the towering and intimidating walls, there is a sense that I am not fully inhabiting my life. I embrace my part as best I can, considering that I have no training on how to be the wife of a prisoner. Reading about grief helps, but then, my story doesn't fit nicely into the formula for reaching what Elizabeth Kubler-Ross describes as "acceptance." I am not a widow. I am only the wife of a man falsely accused who lives in a stone tower.

One year after Phillip's sentence began, I write the following after visiting him in jail:

Voice. It is everything. We could close our eyes and the world would be a song from the breath of each human windpipe of life. I want to close my eyes and listen. Listen to a voice that tells me which way to walk, which path is peace.

There are loud voices in prison, guards joking with each other, yelling directions to visitors, the iron gates electronically opening and closing. The prison cells with bars and no walls, the echo of men's loud voices.

And my husband sitting across from me at the table in the visiting room, his voice is coming from another planet. Not the voice I listened to for eighteen years from beautiful places, from the kitchen table, from the garden, from the front seat of the car, from pillow to pillow.

I want a voice to find me and with my eyes closed I can just listen to this voice tell me anything—tell me about the wind blowing, the fall leaves under the door. Tell me about the planets that are visible and the distance between me and the nearest star. Tell me that what is between the sound of one person and another is more than a breath shaped by the mouth, more than vowels of soft consonants pressing against teeth and palate.

Voices are the only thing I follow when blindfolded by this life that is now mine. I don't want to see the barbed wires, the guards with their nightsticks, and the sergeants with their guns. My husband's spirit is imprisoned. I don't want to see my husband's shaved head, the pain in his eyes, the tears in our daughters' eyes.

There are times when anger exceeds sorrow and rage blinds me. My husband tells me that the guard steals his dinner and if he protests, his telephone privileges are taken away. Or his shower, which he is only entitled to once every three days. He is a forty-six-year-old man who is treated like a child and whose basic needs are subject to the c.o.'s whim. I can feel my heart tightening and something like a small beat of a protest drum flutters against the walls of my chest.

> *My anger takes the form of a bear*
> *night time stars make the shape of a bear*
> *my anger crawls down slowly*
> *(never met it before)*
>
> *eating up the last crumbs*
> *of spontaneous joy.*
> *I deserve a little love, anger says,*
> *I need something that is only mine*
> *hold me!*
> *let me sob*
> *scream*
> *tear the bark off the trees!*
>
> *How angry they have made me*
> *a ferocious*
> *hungry bear.*

The anger and sadness I feel are insurmountable. I channel the feelings into my journal. I never decide in advance what I am going to write nor do I acknowledge my deep mourning until I read what I have written. It is as if I have to jump in to feel that the water is real. As if I don't believe that this is happening to me or to my family. The words bring me in, and at the same time, pull me out. How else can I travel four hours every Tuesday to Green Haven Maximum Security prison to see the man I have been living with and raising a family with for the last eighteen years?

> How can I love the drive to the prison
> the cold hard steps
> the guards who don't greet you kindly
> the metal detectors
> the opening grate of the gate
> the finality of its closing
> the metal dust
> the green and gray dull paint
> the smell of iron flint and aging iron
> my husband's face behind the bars
> his being released into a visiting room
> his long missed hug
> his entering my world for a few hours
> before being taken away
> returning to his 9x6 cell
> living locked away and alone
> without freedom to choose
> what flowers to plant in the garden pots—
> he always planted beautiful flowers.

There are so many different ways to react to a crisis. By now I could have become accustomed to that melting away feeling that a second or third cup of wine brings. I could have continued spending on extravagant wardrobe items. Instead, I call friends at late hours and cry. I indulge in too much chocolate. I yell at the children far more than I would like.

What solace I can't find anywhere else, I find in the blank pages of my journal. It is not one emotion that drives me, but many. Some I cannot name until I have written long enough. Entertaining the grief and providing a place for its anger and sorrow, I am surprised when small points of sun shine through.

I often re-read my journal entries. The words are a labyrinth that I have not figured out how to get through, but I follow my finger over the words as if to find a clue. This is what I wrote one day, when searching for a metaphor that would help me understand my new place in the world:

I have been slung from a slingshot of tragedy into the hemisphere of nothingness—that is what hurts. As if the cord between my husband and my daughters has been severed and each one of us is hurtling out into space in different directions. Some days my heart feels as if it will burn itself out like the end of a wick in a pool of melted wax. Some days Phillip's name is a bone caught in my throat . . .

I experience great empowerment in finding my personal imagery. There is so little control I have right now to change the situation. The structure of justice is complex and, as they say, "The wheels of justice turn slowly." The words, which sometimes grow out of me, are trying to make a connection with a higher spirit or truth.

Time shapes the numbness of shock into a heart full of sorrow. My poet's heart prompts me to find time to be grateful. I want to keep my heart soft and not turn bitter. To keep our home the safe and contained world of warm colored rugs, of simmering onions and garlic, and music playing throughout . . . even if I feel like staying in bed all day, locking the front door, and hiding from the world. There is another page to be written. I am only beginning to understand what my words mean.

The losses of my life push me to go deeper to find my own resilience. I want so much to turn back the hands of time. For the sake of the girls, for my husband, and for myself, I want our family back. More than ever, I feel I must be strong enough to carry everyone across the water on my back.

Like magical thinking, I wish that my writing this story could open the prison gates. After eighteen years of marriage, after all the dreams and intentions of helping the world and raising a loving family are gone, what is left? This is what I am writing to discover.

Phillip, I am building a path, word by word, stone by stone, for you. For you—but also for me. I follow the notebooks, follow the words to a new place.

> *Who knows what purpose*
> *this life? Who knows what reasons*
> *we love, we lose, we suffer,*
> *we live?*
> *And without all this—*
> *a silent rush of emptiness.*
> *We are rich with the stories*
> *of our own arriving.*

Susan's storyline has been stolen. Like a person who returns home to discover a burglary, she tries to make sense of her world. In shock, she sorts the laundry and straightens up magazines. Putting pen to paper is also a way of sorting and imposing order. It is an attempt at mastery and control, having a new go at a reality that is beyond one's comprehension. Her words form a labyrinth, an intricate maze of private passages in an effort to forge a path where none is evident. Susan writes initially for the purpose of absorbing the shock of her husband being accused of molesting his patients.

Susan writes to bear witness to the truth as she knows it. Her truth is in direct conflict with that of the judicial system. In the journal, Susan has the poetic license to express what she cannot voice anyplace else; she vents her grief, her indignation, her anger, and her confusion. The journal is a sanctum—free of wagging tongues and prying eyes. Most importantly, it is a place free of judgment. From her teen years, Susan established the ritual of turning to her journal for self-nurturance and identity affirmation. As she writes, "I had the safety of a lined page in a blank book. I had time to re-read myself until I found the understanding that I wanted from others."

Having the time to "reread myself" is a function of time-shifting. Slowing down to digest her own words helps Susan to integrate thought, feeling, and experience. This expansion of time is especially important when the individual is trying to process a traumatic situation. "There is so little control or power I have right now to change the situation, but in my writings the flow of life experiences is fluid, moving between the past, the present and the future, which is where my hope lies." Time-shifting enables Susan to feel unstuck despite a situation where "time is being served" and life may feel as though it is "on hold."

The intensity of Susan's feelings cannot be contained in ordinary language. The magic of poetic language serves as a highly effective code that simultaneously has the power to contain and release the vast emotions she is experiencing and help her to regulate the emotional intensity through catharsis. "The slingshot of tragedy," "the severed cord," "a heart that will burn itself out like the end of a wick in a pool of melted wax," are all images that capture the violence and collapse of marriage and family life as Susan knew it. Rage is new to her, but she meets it in the form of a grief ravaged bear, "starving for something that is only mine." Metaphor carries multiple levels of meaning and information to both the thinking and feeling parts of the brain; hence, its transformative power.

On a psychological and spiritual level, creativity enables Susan to transcend her limitations. Like an archaeologist, she digs within herself to find new images and juxtapose different ideas. "The words, which sometimes grow out of me, are trying to make a connection with a higher spirit or truth." Her pen is the flashlight in a very dark tunnel. She is writing to attain spiritual awareness and to connect to a Higher Power.

Can the strokes of the pen rewrite the story? Susan has her own story. It is important that this story not be obliterated, or become secondary to her husband's story.

Through writing, she articulates her feelings and thoughts with words that reflect her individuality and identity. Susan's writing is a way for her to hold on to her voice, and not vanish into the supporting role of her husband's drama. Susan, in the act of becoming the story-teller, has the last word as editor of her life. Her words are forming a labyrinth. This web of confusing tunnels and passageways is rich with a story that will ultimately lead to her arrival.

~ 11 ~

The Words That Were Magic Pebbles

Nancy Bengis Friedman

Nancy was in her late twenties when she started to suffer from erratic symptoms that appeared to be unrelated—blindness in one eye, overall weakness, and occasional difficulty walking. It took twelve years to be correctly diagnosed with Multiple Sclerosis (MS).[1] Wheelchair-bound, Nancy's activities became more and more limited. She could no longer perform the activities of daily living—dressing, eating, showering, even urinating—by herself.[2]

However, there was one thing that Nancy could still do. She could write, as long as a scribe was available to take down her words. Despite her helplessness in every other area of her life, when Nancy wrote, she felt empowered. When asked why she writes, Nancy replies, "Writing lets me listen and writing lets me speak."

This is Nancy's story.

DO I HAVE YOUR ATTENTION?

K nowing that someone is listening has always been important to me. As a child, I got attention because of my good grades—a product of my ability to listen well and speak up with the correct answer. I was my parents' pride and joy. I was the best! At least that's what my mother and father told me. Words were my currency, and the objective was love and attention.

If I sound somewhat needy and manipulative, well—I am. When you grow up in a home where your mother rules the roost and your father is a persuasive, high-powered salesman, you become desperate for attention. My father was a Toastmaster; he had joined a brotherhood of dynamic, well-spoken orators who prided themselves on capturing the audience with the spoken word. Mom was a super mom, well-organized, super efficient, and highly directive. So how was I to get a word in edgewise? I wasn't going to compete verbally; instead I became quiet and sardonic. My comments might be few, but they were clever, and writing became a place where I didn't have to compete to get the attention I craved.

My parents were strict and sometimes overbearing, particularly when I reached adolescence. My father made me go out with young men he himself chose—other salesmen's sons. These dates were good for a steak dinner out, but nothing more than that. In high school, I got angry at the girls who were competing with me for boys; they invaded my privacy. Debbie Robinson was my nemesis. She called me a midget one day in front of the school (I'm five-foot-one). Being a polite, and well-bred young lady from the suburbs, I had only one response—"Fuck You!" I cannot tell you the immense satisfaction I had with those two words.

In fact, "Fuck you!" was later to become my mantra. I had pushed down so many years of anger because, when I lived with my parents, anger was unaccepted. I always acquiesced to their wishes. I was a good girl. No, as I said before, the *best* little girl. But all those suppressed fuck-yous had built a wall of resentment inside. By the time I was twenty-one, the face I showed the world was sweet, cute, and calm, but inside a volcano was brewing.

My therapist at that time gave me the perfect solution to shattering my "good girl myth." Whenever anyone said or did anything that upset me, they received a "Fuck You!" that was inevitably met with surprise, shock, and sometimes delight. Of course I never said this to my parents. My f-you tool was one of the best things that ever happened to me. Armed with these two words, I was ready to take on the world. Until I became a respectable married lady.

I met a young man named Bob Friedman one fortuitous day in a Park Avenue doctor's office. He was thirty-five but had a boyish grin and charmed me completely. We were married within a year, and we had our first son one year later. Little Jedediah had a brother, Seth, four years later. I found family life challenging, but I loved my boys dearly. I couldn't have been happier. I never suspected the challenge ahead of me.

THE DISEASE

For several years, I experienced strange symptoms that departed as mysteriously as they arrived. The occasional twitching and muscle weakness were annoying symptoms, but the doctors reassured me it was nothing to worry about. But by the time I was in my late thirties, I lost the ability to feel certain things. My senses seemed dulled. My world blurred. I lost the ability to control my urine. I had to be catheterized twice a day. I felt like a baby. I felt stupid—I, who had always prided myself on being smart and mature.

What was this demon that had taken over my body? When I couldn't walk, and at one point couldn't see, I still couldn't believe it. It must be a cosmic trick. God must be playing a trick on me. Hadn't I been a good girl? No, even the best girl of all. I did once cheat on a test. That must be the reason. Or, perhaps I told a white lie or two. But this kind of punishment? Impossible.

After ten years of misdiagnoses, I learned the name of this strange beast—Multiple Sclerosis. Many years went by before I was able to write the following poem, "What MS Might Be":

Perhaps it's a snake with tiny teeth
nibbling away at my nerve endings.
Green, a garden snake with tiny teeth,
Or perhaps it's a memory lost,
A night that happened long ago that
Flashes before me
A memory fading and returning . . .
No, perhaps MS is a fantasy in which I am raped.
I hear your voice saying, "You'll never remember this."
Ha! I do remember.
This is MS—a snake, a thief, a rapist.
I must stomp on the snake.
I must testify against the thief.
I must escape the rapist.
And somehow I must become the victor.

Multiple Sclerosis took over every aspect of my life. My role as wife and mother was supplanted; the disease took over. My children would not come home to June Cleaver baking cookies in the afternoon. My husband would not come home to Betty Crocker's cooking. The refrigerator was empty. The house was not an advertisement for Better Homes and Gardens.

But I still wanted to be listened to and respected and admired. Even better, to be worshipped as an icon (just kidding!). In my previous life, I had been respected as a teacher, writer, and poet. But now, my memory was shot. The disease was robbing me of my balance, physically, creatively, and mentally.

BEST FRIENDS

I can't cry anymore—except into my writing journal. My eyes don't produce tears. Ironic, isn't it? The journal is the avenue for tears, laughter, regression, irony, and whatever else I may be feeling. It becomes a nonjudgmental space I can go to at anytime. I can write down my complaints, my fears, and my regrets without feeling like a crybaby.

With whom can I share my life? My old friends are busy with their own lives. I sit confined, unable to get myself up, dust myself off, and start all over again. Don't we take it all for granted when we are healthy? But here I was, day after day, alone except for . . . words, my daily visitors, my best friends.

Best Friends

What? Words?
They are my best friends,
Always available, never spiteful,
Sometimes clever, sometimes ironic,
Sometimes piercing.
To what end?
Words are spilling, tumbling, sauntering
Dancing their way onto the page,
They will seduce you,
You must buy them, enjoy them,
Show them off to other friends,
Ones you haven't seen in a while.
They'll remember
The prize, the wonder, the thrill.
Why?
'Cuz I say so!
Got a problem with it?
Got a word? Add an s—it's a sword!
I can fight with words,
I can sell with words,
I can love with words . . .
Stay tuned.

Life is damn boring when day after day you are unable to leave your home. I have to imagine alternative possibilities and create drama. No problem. Why? Because I've got words, and words will create their own adventures. My adventures—created consciously or unconsciously—shake me up, shock me, and thrill me. Creating adventure through my imagination provides me with stimulation. My imagination can be fed by a word, an image, or any interaction with something in my environment.

A Poem Can Strike
A poem can strike
at the oddest moments.
It can be an obituary
in The New York Times,
an obituary about the sudden
death of a novelist
whose work you'd been devouring
for months,

or the sight eye to eye
of a lobster in a tank,
claws chained and yet gazing at you
with a wisdom so human
you knew it had
to live in a poem,

or the poem could be born in the darkness
of an Amtrack Silver Star
bumping and roaring down the eastern Seaboard,
its riders, a carnival.

It could be the seventy-nine-year-old dentist
who called himself "Lightning"
and despised the rubber gloves
they demand he wear
whenever he explored an open mouth
for cavities.

A poem can ask to be born
in the old woman pacing
back and forth
in the train,
her hair crimped beneath
a pink triangle
of cotton.
She never said a word.
A poem can strike
at the oddest moments.

Without my imagination, I would be desperate, sad, and pathetic. Instead, I choose the role of Athena, the goddess of wisdom, the Queen Kahuna and all the heroic characters who conquer and triumph over every obstacle.[3]

Chutzpah!

I can do anything—
Just give me a wall to hang onto,
a wall and a banister to guide me.
Up, down, east or west—
Anywhere is possible.
I'll try it, crawling, like Spider-Woman,
or tumbling like Zena, somersaulting,
with the warrior's cry.
Always landing on my feet,
Always getting what I want when I want it.
Maybe enjoying a gentleman's hand
well-offered and well-placed.
I admit to vulnerability.
There are moments when I am powerless
*   to do anything.*
I consider it a stroke of fate that puts me in a position

where I cannot move,
but then I'm struck by the power of counting from one to ten
in Yiddish, in Spanish and in French.
And then it comes over me—
I hear my father's voice saying, "You can do anything, Nancy B.,
If you put your mind to it. I've seen you do it before. One thing we
Bengises have always had—the nerve."
Nerve?
A wall, a banister, and one essential ingredient—CHUTZPAH!

Despite my love affair with the heroine's journey, there are still times when—pardon my French—life sucks. Life feels hopeless, bleak, and barren —a desert of nothingness. I know that there's meaning out there . . . my meaning. I cannot tolerate the superficiality. I must create the meaning out of nothing. Shall we turn straw into gold? Shall we have another cup of coffee? A raisin cookie perhaps?

I told my mother-in-law, Sylvia, "It all sucks."

She replied, "Write another poem." I repeated it louder this time. "It all sucks."

And she said, "You have to be stronger than that."

"It all *fucking* sucks."

She said, "That's better."

I think of better times, when I was stronger, and the old fuck-you-ness of me was alive and kicking. I need to reclaim it, but it seems to elude me . . . the old fuck-you-ness of me was a sweet thing. I miss it.

A Pretty Thing
The old fuck-you-ness of me
was a pretty thing
a nasty thing
a don't mess with me kind of thing.
So cool . . . so powerful.
I loved her and her in your faceness.

Where did she go?
I think delivering a baby
knocked me down
with a one two punch
Then getting a disease which
knocked me down
another few notches
to be redeemed now by
another kind of bravura,
a new kind of toughness—
a kind that doesn't cry,
that keeps a tough upper lip,
that gets a new kind of admiration,
but this time it's mixed with pity,
not high fives and a nod of
recognition.
I miss the old fuck-you-ness of me
and need to try boxing lessons
to feel the chutzpa's back.

WHO CARES?

At one point my intense loneliness and need for attention led me to become friendly with any telemarketer who called. However, by the time I verbally committed myself to a timeshare in Florida, a cubic zirconia ring, and a set of Encyclopedia Britannica, my husband was fit to be tied and banned me from the computer and phone. Looking back at that time in my life, I see the acute irony and humor in this situation. Dom de Luise had the same problem of getting sucked into a sales pitch. Or was it the salesperson who got sucked into my agenda? I kept them talking. They asked me questions about my life, and I was happy to have some company for a few minutes. They made a sale, and I was flattered by the attention. So what if we had different agendas? As for the credit card bills, well, that was another matter. My husband eventually took my credit cards away from me, putting an end to my mischief.

There are days when I feel abandoned, sad, angry, frustrated, and pathetic. And I wonder, "Who cares?" The world keeps turning. My family and friends go about their business. And I sit, confined. At those moments, my house turns into a prison, and I long for escape. The young, adventurous girl in me still wants to be a key player, a star in the limelight, an important somebody. And so the childhood desire for attention that my parents instilled and fed continues. Does anyone really care?

Who Cares About Nancy?

Who cares about Nancy?
Who cares if she's happy or inspired,
whether she's hostile or peaceful?
What difference does it make to anyone?
Of course it should make a difference to Nancy herself.

Perhaps I can find the magic
in the silence,
in the quiet.
I am searching for
a spark to ignite
the fire inside.
The tinder of my imagination
can become a raging flame.
O' spirit, rise to the possibility
of creation.
Summon me to write.
I stand freezing where the winds blow mightily.
Dare I escape the house
and enter the world beyond my door
to follow a path
all my own?

This need for attention works for me and against me at the same time. Every minute of attention feeds the cookie monster, who is so hungry for attention. But when cookie monster doesn't get attention, my addictive tendencies emerge. I hunt frenetically for attention, or I have symptoms of withdrawal. On the other hand, when the cookie monster gets too filled with attention, indigestion follows.

Truthfully, my need for attention has only gotten worse with my disease. The fact that I am pale, petite, and appear to be in need of attention only encourages this cookie monster behavior. As an invalid, I find people are very sympathetic, and for a while, I played this for all it was worth. For example, one day, when I was outside the house and still able to walk on my own, I fell and got quite a lot of attention on the street. Several people came over to me and formed a huddle, wondering what they could do for me. I could not help but feel a flush of pleasure at this attentiveness. I continued to periodically spend time outside my home, and people who remembered my collapsing would come over, asking how I was.

As my symptoms got worse, my role as mother, housekeeper, and wife was challenged. Perhaps worst of all, I had to relinquish my professional status and identity as a teacher. I was sad. I missed the students. I hungered for the attentiveness and responsiveness, which gave me such pleasure. What could be more pleasurable than writing a reference for a young person applying for college and setting out into the world? I missed this world, and with its loss I felt a tremendous void.

Many of my writings deal with this void. In one of my poems, I compare myself to a cracked, porcelain vase:

> Orchids once lived here, purple and lush,
> and the vase you see before you
> is empty and hoping to be filled.

The leaking vase image appears again in the following poem:

Worthlessness
My worthlessness is the worthlessness of
    a leaking vase
an empty dish
    a bed with no one in it
a cloud with no rain to fall
    a tv with no source of power
a scissor with one blade
It's all useless
    pointless
It makes me cry without tears
because my body no longer produces tears . . .
Is it an age thing?
Is it an MS thing?
Me with eyes that cannot cry,
legs that walk only small distances.
How shall I measure the cup of self-worth?
Right now I'm very thirsty.

There are days when I feel very much the victim. The MS demon has a family of smaller demons. I feel helpless and I cannot count on my ability to do anything. For example, just walking across a room cannot be done alone. Peeing cannot be accomplished by oneself. When one is confronted daily by so many tasks one cannot do without help, a daunting sense of worthlessness haunts the victim. The simplest functions of the body that we take for granted become huge.

To Pee or Not to Pee—That Is the Question . . .
Does the sun come up each morning
    and go down at dusk?
It was never a question till now—
It was never such a big deal before this

211

I have to be prepared every day
wear protective pads
but I also need assistance from my husband,
        who writes me love letters with the tip of the catheter
twice a day
No other lovemaking between us
except for this intimate gesture
this translucent tubing
extracting a golden stream of fluid
        waste
    precious gold
because it brings him closer to me.

For a time, along with other medications, I was receiving testosterone shots. When under the influence of these testosterone shots, I felt
speedy, powerful, and wanted to take on the world. I actually became high
for a week or two. But then the descent would take place. I would crash. I
became depressed and hopeless. I wrote this when I was at an all time low.

Ready for the Knife
my eyes fasten on
a bottle of olive oil
a silent dishwasher
an empty oven
four bananas lie calmly
ready for the knife that will cut them into pieces
it is a busy kitchen, a full kitchen,
the signs of life everywhere—
dishes for eating,
mother, father, brother, brother,
my mother, his mother, just a phone call away.
it is a beige phone with a long cord
good for long distance conversations.

I miss the intimacy and immediacy of life mattering.
my eyes fasten on
a bottle of olive oil
a silent dishwasher
an empty oven
four bananas lie calmly
ready for the knife that will cut them into pieces . . .

Fortunately, we soon realized that the testosterone shots were causing these mood swings, and I discontinued them. The suicidal feelings stopped. The bad feelings went away. However, as I became physically weaker and weaker, I depended more and more on the people around me. An aide was hired to assist me on a daily basis. I felt my authority dwindle away. My mother, my husband, my sons, and my aide all seemed to make decisions for me and thought they knew what was in my best interests.

As my little self was growing smaller and smaller, I struggled to maintain a sense of autonomy and authority. Aides who were bossy or dominating did not last long. I struggled and still struggle with this issue. Who is in charge? Is the aide working for me, or vice versa? If she's working for me, why do I feel like I'm taking orders?

Labor Relationships
Bob said a clever thing I must remember.
Don't let an employee undermine you,
cuz after all,
Who is the boss?
I forgot the power of that phrase.
Who is the boss?
By golly,
Who is the boss???
Me!

Magic Pebbles under My Tongue

Neediness is not a pretty feeling. I don't ever want to be a burden on my family. This is a demon I don't usually acknowledge. It thrives on my feelings of worthlessness. Our family lives by the eleventh commandment: DO NOT BE SELFISH! This commandment is "Put aside your selfish desires," particularly if they interfere with the desires of another. The "other" is a) your husband, b) your sons, c) your mother, and last on the list, as always, d) myself. These omniscient judges, juries, and panels sit ever ready to take me down. Of course, I am the worst judge and jury is of all.

What happens when the family wants to go out to a special event that does not accommodate my wheelchair? Am I left behind? Do I stop them from going? Do I make my needs known? How do I balance my needs with theirs? This is an ongoing battle.

I am always trying to mediate my needs for attention, for companionship, and stimulation.[4] Writing and reading my work to other people helps me to fill the void. There is a special relationship between writers and readers. The knowledge that you will be heard and responded to is intrinsic to the relationship. We choose those we have a relationship with, and we can enjoy or suffer with our choices. It gives me happiness to know that you, who are reading this, at this very moment, will listen to my words and know me in some way. After all, we are in a relationship. This is on a good day.

Occasionally I still feel infantilized and dependent because I need so much assistance. But most of the time I feel content. My attitude of gratitude for life's small and great blessings returned. I am thankful for the constancy and predictability of all the people in my life—from the New York Police Department and firemen who stand by, to my mother, my sister, my aide, my therapist, and my immediate family, who are my greatest champions.

Anything that can be depended on
is a thing to be loved,
as I depend on you, Bob, my husband

214

and Jed, my son, and Seth, my son.
I depend on you—not to do anything,
but to be loving in my world.
Simply to be there,
like the sun in the sky,
like the moon and the stars;
not always visible but always returning
Returning to me.

When I get too quiet or depressed, my therapist reminds me of the importance of my "magic pebbles." My words exist like magic pebbles waiting under my tongue to be spoken. Writing has been, from the beginning, my way of expressing my point of view and my way of being in the world. I'm a very small person who needs to get beyond her size to get out into the world. My words, like magic pebbles, are now unlodged from beneath my tongue. May the pebbles roll and be discovered by you.

Words have become Nancy's best friends. They reduce the isolation in her life, and keep her company. The page is listening like an understanding friend. Nancy is both sender and receiver in the communication process. Part of the self is writing; part of the self is reading and observing. This enables Nancy to experience more fully her thoughts and feelings. She is reclaiming fragments of herself and using her creativity to integrate parts into the whole. This is extremely important because Nancy suffers from severe memory loss (a frequent symptom of multiple sclerosis), resulting in a general sense of loss and confusion. A poem in black and white gives Nancy a sense of clarity, security, and capability. In addition, the poems can be shared, and word-gifts facilitate socialization.

Nancy's illness poses challenges to her identity: "As my little self was growing smaller and smaller, I struggled to maintain a sense of autonomy and authority." With the exacerbation of symptoms and increasing disability, she states, "My worthlessness is the worthlessness of a leaking vase." She writes poignantly about missing her professional identity: "Orchids once lived here, purple and lush, / and the vase you see before you / is empty and waiting to be filled."

Although Nancy feels diminished and incapacitated, she is still capable of creating a poem. The poem provides concrete proof of her productivity and bolsters her ego. Most importantly it is a reclaiming of voice and a unique signature of personality. When Nancy uses her voice to express her thoughts and feelings, she is an active person who can impact others; when she stops using her voice, she becomes a passive, non-participant who feels objectified and infantilized in the world.

Being unable to hold a pen has not stopped Nancy from expressing herself. Many of Nancy's poems were written during the past fifteen years in therapy with Dr. Reiter. Nancy dictated the lines to her therapist, who sat at the computer, typing her words. Nancy is proud, and not one to show much emotion to others. However, her journal is a safe container that holds all of her emotions without reprisal. She writes, "I can't cry anymore . . . The journal is the avenue for tears . . . I can write down my complaints, my fears, and my regrets without feeling like a crybaby." Nancy's poetic license grants her permission to vent, and is vital to her sense of well-being.

The magic of the poetic enhances Nancy's sense of freedom and safety and empowers her to write about topics that are taboo. Urine becomes "precious gold"—transformation of matter—because her daily catheterization brings her husband closer to her. In "Ready for the Knife," Nancy uses poetic device to capture the depersonalization and a feeling of dissociation that she is experiencing during a severe depression. "The four bananas lie calmly ready for the knife that will cut them to pieces." Nancy is able to transform time, space, and matter with metaphor. The knife is symbolic of the self-destructive anger, and the four bananas may signify the four members of Nancy's family.

"Ready for the Knife" was instrumental in identifying Nancy's suicidal ideation at a time when she experienced a counter-therapeutic

216

reaction to medication. In this case, the poem became a red flag for the therapist, who then alerted the family to expedite appropriate medical care. Sometimes a poem is like an emotional x-ray, and in the clinician's hands, it may be used diagnostically.

In summary, Nancy's writing reflects five purposes of therapeutic writing: 1. for nurturance and self-affirmation; 2. for self-regulation of emotion ("I don't have a way to cry—except into my writing journal"); 3. for clarity and organization; 4. for integration; and 5. for stimulation ("I've got words, and words will create their own adventures").

Nancy may become physically weaker, but as long as she has the power to dip into her expressive imagination and reclaim her voice, her psychological health will remain intact.

Nancy writes, "I'm a very small person, who needs to get beyond her size to get out into the world." Writing gives Nancy a sense of empowerment and mastery. The words, like magic pebbles, roll from her tongue into the greater world, and suddenly she is not so small.

~ 12 ~

Notes from the Back of the Class
Mark Auster

John Keats once wrote, "The imagination of a boy is healthy, and the mature imagination of a man is healthy; but there is a space in the life between, in which the soul is in a ferment, the character undecided, the way of life uncertain, the ambition thick-sighted . . ."[1] Adolescence can be a challenging time of physical and emotional changes, raging hormones, and peer pressure. Erikson called this phase between childhood and adulthood "identity vs. identity confusion."[2] It is a transitional time that often includes experimentation with different behaviors and values in order to discover the true self.

For Mark Auster, it is particularly tumultuous. His mother has a chronic illness and his father is rarely at home. In addition to dealing with the social scene, and a desperate striving for popularity, he is coping with depression,[3] mood swings, and social anxiety. School is a day-to-day struggle. Relationships are difficult. Mark has already discovered marijuana and alcohol; they take the edge off the tension he feels. More than anything, Mark craves acceptance and social status. But first he will need to learn to accept himself. And in the process, he will discover his true identity.

This is Mark's story. _____

TO TELL THE TRUTH

Notebook Entry—February 23, 2002

    I confess it now. I am a liar. I am manipulative, self-centered, and I make no excuse for what I'm doing (cutting class, smoking weed for the third day in a row). It's definitely not the right decision for most. It's unrealistic, irresponsible, and just plain stupid. Mainly because I'm not giving myself a chance to experience what life has to offer. But what does life have to offer anyway? Disappointment, rejection, evil people who betray and backstab you the first chance they get. Frankly, this life doesn't seem all that appealing to me. Of course, who am I to argue the age-old question: To be or not to be? Well, let's review my qualifications.

    Almost twenty years of life experience, most of it spent watching TV and movies, playing video games, staring at a computer; basically I've spent most of the best years of my life staring at a screen of pixels. I guess that's not experience at all. I've never had sex. I've never known the love of a girl although I've been infatuated with many. Sadly, the fact is that my experience carries no real weight. The only thing that keeps me going is the possibility that things could change. After all, the next sixty some odd years do have quite a bit of potential. I just have to get out of the current rut. Unfortunately, it's a deep rut that I've been in—for a long time.

This journal entry was written six years ago, when I was nineteen. I'm twenty-four, but I floundered in a rut for about eight years, starting at age sixteen. I needed some help getting out of it. That was part of my problem. I just didn't know how to ask for help. Instead I would try to do it by myself, feel myself fail, and just give up. It's a cycle. I fall into a depressed mood.[2] I withdraw from relationships and commitments. The cell phone becomes an object that I fear. Unread voice mails pile up. Eventually, I am so overwhelmed that I don't even answer the phone. During this time, moods swing from high to low. When I'm up, I feel great, but my feelings may plummet quickly. All it takes is failing a test or not being able to rise to a social situation. The failures pile on one another, snowballing into deep depression.

Ups and Downs

Emotions sway me like a young tree in a storm
I must not allow my trunk to hold too stiff
Only by swaying can I hope to not snap
Tsunamis of sadness, fear and yearning
They crash over my huddling mortal soul
I coil into a ball and only hope to survive
Yet the wave does pass eventually
I am left to dry and wait for the next battle
I will hold my sword and wait
In the time in between, let's see what I can accomplish.

The time between tsunamis was when I would get my act together. I was able to function well in that in-between period, but it never lasted. Were my ups and downs caused by a chemical flaw in my make-up or was it my environment? Maybe it was both.

To make matters worse, I suffered from social anxiety. When a pretty girl was near me, I became self-conscious and an internal dialogue began. It would go something like this: "She looks uncomfortable. I'd like to make physical contact to let her know I want to connect. But is it appropriate? Or will I scare her off? These pauses are painful. I'll fill in the silences. Oh, no, I said something stupid. Now I'm even more self-conscious! Damn it. Now I've blown it." My self-consciousness was not restricted to girls. When I didn't feel good about myself, I was just as awkward with the guys. For most of my life, all I wanted was to be part of the in crowd . . . acceptance in the golden circle.

IN AND OUT OF THE CLIQUE

Social status has always been paramount in my personal value system. As far back as I can remember, even in kindergarten, people made fun of me. They called me "Forgetful Jones" because I would forget my hat in the lunchroom or leave a book at home that I was supposed to bring to class. Even then I was absent-minded—as I am now. So there was a desire not to be singled out in ridicule. At age five, I was intent on impressing those around me and sought recognition with grandiose stories. I told my first lie in kindergarten, when I boasted to my teacher that I had just come back from France. (Imagine my parents' reaction, when, during parent-teacher conference, the teacher exclaimed how wonderful it was that I had been exposed to a foreign country at such a young age; of course they had no idea what she was talking about).

My lies became more elaborate over time. By age nine, I told my schoolmates there was a secret passage in my room. It was a hidden door that led to a paradise of video games and toys. All my classmates wanted to go home with me. I actually did have a small door that led nowhere, and when friends came to visit, I made up an excuse that it wasn't the right time to enter the treasure trove. It became second nature for me to lie.

The problem was that I tried to be someone that I'm not. That has been the foundation for a great deal of mental turmoil. Because status has been a high priority, I've been slow to learn how to love people. Love requires stepping out of one's own desires, focusing on someone else. I have only recently come to understand that there needs to be a balance between the energy spent on self and energy spent on others. I think that my problems started with an unhealthy preoccupation of self and what others think of me.

In elementary school and junior high, I mostly hung out with my best friend, Josh, who was chubby. There was a group of cool kids; they were sexually active, experimented with drugs and alcohol, and broke the rules. And miracle of miracles, in the eighth grade they gravitated toward me. I somehow fulfilled their requirements. They considered me good-looking, athletic, funny, and personable. So, I ditched my chubby, un-cool friend, Josh, in a heartbeat. I loved Josh, but he was a liability to my new social status. I ended up in the cool crowd, drinking and smoking. (Sorry, Josh, I was a lousy friend). I deeply regret that I squandered a potentially life-long friendship.

By now I was a proficient liar. Maybe the truth just isn't impressive enough, so I spice it up. I don't want to say I'm a virgin so I say, oh, yeah, I've slept with five or six women. If I failed a class, hey—I got an A! I even lied about small, inconsequential things. (Did you do your homework? Sure, Dad). I saw no harm in telling other people what they wanted to hear. I tried to be whomever the other person wanted me to be. Later, I started to lie to my friends when depression or social anxiety kept me from socializing. I didn't understand that the core of friendship is honesty. I thought the core was impressing others. I lied to my friends, my parents, my teachers, and of course, myself.

LIAR

I'm a liar
Sometimes I'm sad
I'm a liar
Sometimes I'm glad
I'm a liar
Sometimes I deceive my friends
I'm a liar
I'm hard to offend
I'm a liar
Take me or leave me
I'm a liar
I live in a grey sea
I'm a liar
Is it bad?
I'm a liar
Some call me a rad
I'm a liar
no one knows
I'm a liar
it festers and grows
nobody understands
I don't let them
I am a Rhino, a solitary creature

I reach out but I cut myself off
I can't focus
I want to cry
No tears come
I stare into others eyes
I can't stop saying I, I, I, I, I, I, I
Someone else (just felt like breaking up the monotony)
I is very monotonous, such is the inner dialogue
My mother asks me, "Who do you love?" I have no answer
I am alone

My difficulties started in high school. I went to a school for the gifted and the academic competition was keen. In the last year, my grades went down. I experimented with pot and alcohol. I had a tremendous desire to be a party animal, to be able to talk with the girls, and hang out with the guys. I seemed to fit in, but there was a part of me that was always observing the group, analyzing them from the outside, a part of me that was separate and alone.

On the home front, my mom, the person I felt closest to, was sick and getting worse. I had watched my mother's slow deterioration from a neurological disease over the past decade. As my mother's condition worsened, my father withdrew as an active presence at home. I spent time with Mom, who needed a little help sometimes because she was unsteady. At first it wasn't so bad. She could walk with a cane. She fell occasionally, but she still functioned—up until the time she burned herself. I was a junior in high school at the time. She was in the Cornell Hospital Burn Unit for four months.

I remember going to and from the hospital in a detached, numb way as though it was all happening to someone else. It was surreal, like a nightmare. It seemed crazy that my mother was bedridden in a hospital, refusing to eat. I can easily recall vivid images of the hospital food that my mother refused to eat— the look of covered trays, the smell of hospital food, the red jello that remained untouched. When she came back from the hospital, she couldn't walk and was in a wheelchair. It hurt to see her like that. I couldn't look at her, so I avoided her. No one talked about it. I had to deal with it on my own. I took the intense anxiety I felt and channeled it toward the social circle.

Perhaps this was the beginning of my social anxiety. I just wanted to fit in. But even in elementary school I knew our family was different. I avoided bringing friends back to the house. There was never any food in the house. Dad was away most of the time, running his company; when he was home I got into power struggles with him. It was not my mother's fault that she could not be fully present, but what about my father? His absence was inexcusable! Inside me a black rage began to bubble. In a sense, I had no parents, and no home—at least not like a normal family.

My rage was tempered with grief. Why did this have to happen to my Mom? Why did she have to suffer? I witnessed the slow transformation of my mother into an invalid, and I felt helpless. I could not change the situation, so I tried to blot it out. Smoking marijuana helped. No one was there to watch me, monitor me, or reign me in.

It was around this unhappy time that I started writing. Somehow the empty page was a comfort to me. Instead of listening to the drone of the teacher in class, I wrote:

> The empty page sits in front of me
> It is in the lotus position—a peaceful Buddha
> I destroy its balance with my thoughts
> My pen hovers over the page
> I am holding back
> Why must I filter the flow
> The pitcher that is my mind—arm, hand, fingers—
> Only wishes to pour freely
> A thick, luscious liquid
> Ecstasy and fear all in one
> My skin pours on the verge of explosion
> My whole being only wishes to secrete feelings . . .

Writing was a place to go when I felt trapped. It became a refuge for me, where I could release my emotions. It was the place I never lied. My notebooks are filled with my personal writing. It was hard to focus in class. My mind seemed to be running in place.

Notebook Entry— January 5, 2003

>*She sits to my right, a kindred spirit. Talk to her, sit next to her, for God's sake.*
>
>*Fear paralyzes me. A transient emotion that passes through me like wind through the fall leaves that litter the streets; they are tired and wrinkled, like my diminished self-confidence. I remain, cramped in a wooden school chair, yearning, hoping that my fear will not dominate me. I feel trapped. My mind races with no end, fragmented. Unintelligent at times, it toils through futility. A scrap of a pop song, a flash of sexual fantasy, a memory from elementary school. Why do these random synapses fire off in the manner they do? What I seek is order. I desire logic and machine-like analytical ability. If only I could rope in the excess thoughts and filter out the unnecessary chaff . . .*

In my last year of high school, I could no longer concentrate on academics. Grades went down and colleges rescinded their acceptances. I became aloof socially and felt depressed. I started smoking pot by myself. It was the ultimate indulgence. When I smoked, the mundane became enjoyable. I could watch TV and, because of the smoking, I felt serene and content. If you're high, you can build a fantasy life easily. It fed my emotional needs and destroyed my social skills. Eventually a heavy depression settled in.

I plodded through summer school, graduated high school, and finally went off to SUNY Albany. I made a strong effort to succeed. At first I was doing well. But then I missed an assignment. Each successive failure to perform led me to a landslide of anxiety and depression. One morning I just did not want to get out of bed. Not that morning or the morning after. What could I say? That it was hard for me to get out of bed? Sounds lame, doesn't it? But it was the truth. I felt paralyzed, exhausted and depressed. I could not face the day. I could not face other people. So yes, the inevitable happened.

I flunked out, and returned home shamefaced and without explanation.

Eventually, I got into a community college. (Of course I lied to my friends, who thought I was still attending SUNY). My father insisted that I get a degree. And when I was not thinking the worst of myself, I wanted a degree also. I loved philosophy, politics, and literature. I liked nothing better than an intellectual discussion. However, I did not like going to school. Although certain courses and teachers were interesting, I found most of the courses boring. They weren't too difficult for me. They were usually too easy. I just didn't bother to do the work, and then at midterms and finals I had to cram and jump through hoops. I tried to take notes in each class, but my internal world dominated. Here's a typical entry made during Physics Class:

Notebook Entry— April 16, 2003
Mostly Nitrogen
A large room full of people surrounds me. Many are engaged in dialogue. I sit, iso-
lated. A feeling of anxiety surges from my groin through my torso. The conversa-
tions end as the teacher tries to draw the students' attention back to the lesson.
Most are not listening. Some do so only out of obligation. The classroom is sup-
posed to be an energized sanctuary, a place where wisdom is imparted. This would
not be how I describe my surroundings. One hundred or so wooden chairs,
arranged in stadium style seating. Half are filled with the warm bodies of students.
The teacher's heavy Korean accent obscures his words. I wonder if, during his
pauses, he is thinking in his native language or English . . .

Socially, I would go out, get high and become uncontrollably anx-ious. I would experience paralysis if someone looked at me the wrong way. I obsessed about how I was viewed in others eyes—my clothes, my speech, my image. I was deeply preoccupied by what others thought of me. I fixated on girls. I wanted to touch and kiss them, but I couldn't even start a conversa-tion. It was a scenario that was to repeat itself over and over during my col-lege years when I went to bars and parties.

Then there were times when I tried to fake it. My cousin, a popular yuppie, took me to a fancy bar. I was surrounded by beautiful people. I talked the talk, and anyone watching would have thought I was having a good time, but inside I was terrified. There was no correlation between what I felt inside—pure animal fear—and my external loquacious behavior. But fear took over; I felt as though I were being preyed upon. I fled the bar without saying good-bye to my cousin. I saw myself as a cowardly rabbit, either frozen or on the run. I wrote a series of rabbit poems. This is one of them:

> *Billions upon billions of atomic particles separate us*
> *Me and my soul mate*
> *My desire*
> *Who?*
> *To stare and yearn is worthless*
> *The salvation of paper and pen*
> *Fear that paralyzes me from so much as eye contact*
> *I am a rabbit*
> *My forest is endless*
> *Yet I do not roam beyond my small enclave*
> *But I have my endless imagination as my*
> *Retreat*

Obsessed with my sense of failure. I accused myself of the worst possible inadequacy and felt deep self-hatred. All the other guys were able to do it. I saw them approach pretty girls with success. I wanted to talk to them too. It tore me up inside. I was fiercely jealous and hated my own ineptness. My moods vacillated. When I was feeling good, I had confidence, but when depression took over, in the depths of my belly, I was a queasy, self-conscious mess, oozing doubt and fear.

Internal Struggle
> *Two forces at battle within*
> *I own both of them*
> *They are dual incarnations of my spirit*

One resides in the depths of my belly
The other rests atop my proud shoulders
The belly dweller is a nasty fellow
He feeds on my fears and self-doubts
I have fed him well over the years
The by-product of the belly dweller is anxiety
A bubbling, crackling vat of self-doubt . . .

These two aspects of self were tearing me apart. I tried to stay on even keel, neither too high nor too low. I tried to fill my hours by working part-time so as not to fall back into watching TV and smoking marijuana. But inevitably the anxiety would get to me. I repeatedly failed courses, and repeatedly lied. I broke appointments with friends, and lied some more. I moved in the fog of marijuana, submerged in self-pity and fear. I felt only half alive.

THERAPY

My parents insisted I go to therapy when I was about eighteen. I went to the first therapist and promptly sabotaged the process by lying to him. I went two or three times and then refused to go back to him. The second therapist was Dr. Reiter; I felt I could talk to this therapist, and she didn't seem to judge me. I felt an immediate connection to Dr. Reiter, but occasionally I lied to her too. Nevertheless, therapy was the place I could ask my questions, and I had a lot of them.

Identity
Who am I? Where do I stand?
So many paths close at hand
My time has come to step up to the plate
Will I swing and miss? Will I wait?
Of course success is to what I aspire
But what is success, what is my desire?

228

Loads of money, surely happiness will follow
Greed and Lust is where I can wallow
Yet tired I will grow of Flesh and Toys
So where must I look? Where is my joy?
Religion, ahhh . . . God will save me
Study the Talmud or the Bible maybe?
Are these the answers for which I look
Ink or paper, pages in a book?
My entire life, these questions I will ask
Never answers—Asking is my task.

There were, of course, questions I dared not ask. I pushed certain questions away, but they surfaced periodically. What would happen to my mother? Where did my father go Saturday nights, and why did he come back in the early hours of the morning? My hunch was that he was having an affair. But who knew? Frankly, I didn't really want to know. Most of my questions were about my self. Was my fear of success greater than my need to succeed? Why was it so difficult for me to talk to girls? Was I gay? Bisexual? Such thoughts swirled inside me. Meanwhile, I continued to smoke pot. I knew that the pot might be affecting my motivation. I knew that alcohol was a depressant. But I felt I had no other weapons to fight the pain of the depression and anxiety.

Trapped and in limbo, I lived inside my head, muttering internal dialogues. I wrote poems to a girl I never spoke to. I got so used to talking to myself, it was frightening. I was often filled with self-hatred, confusion, and anger. My pen was my only weapon, and my paper became a confidante. Unspoken feelings and urges spiraled inside me, tangled and confused. Through writing I would net these submerged thoughts and feelings, refining them into fine sand. I filled up my mind and body with bags of sand, and provided bandages for the holes in my soul, seeping existential fear and anxiety.

229

My work is always lost
Even before it is written
What am I?
I feel
I think
What is my goal?
Do I want to be Ken Wilbur or Zbigniew Brezinski?
Can I be either?
Is it worth it to try?
What is beyond a question? Is an answer anything more than death?
It is a beautiful day today. Why am I crying?

Therapy continued to be a safe place for me to express my feelings. My therapist taught me cognitive therapy techniques, and I worked on replacing my self-denigrating statements with more positive ones. Sometimes it worked; sometimes it didn't. I expressed my anger and sadness through role play. Occasionally I would bring in a poem I had written for discussion. In my last year of therapy, I wrote a poem about my mother that was extremely significant:

I see you collapsing, falling, wrenching with pain
Take me instead, oh God
Why does she have to be the martyr?
I yearn to relieve your pain
If your destiny is this, then I will join you in it
We will be partners in pain—
But no, this strategy only leads me to sadness and anger
It only allows a vicious cycle to continue
This is not what you would want for me
I must draw strength from your struggle
You are a warrior, an Olympian, a hero
You have filled my soul with wisdom
The wisdom of strength and perseverance

Perseverance to deal with both sides of life
The beauty and the joy—but also the fear and the setbacks
The demons within me are strong
Still, the sword with which I will fight them was forged
By your wisdom and strength
Let's fight together.

This poem represents a turning point in my therapy. I was able to articulate something that I could not previously say. The poem suggests that I had joined my mother by taking on a depressed, apathetic persona. It was not something that I had done consciously. But I identified with my mother strongly. We both wrote poetry. We both told little lies on occasion. When she was healthy, she had been a great storyteller. (I like nothing better than a good story). There was an unspoken bond between us. Illness had left her a shell of what she had originally been. For me, it was a profound, ongoing loss.

In addition to individual therapy, my mother, father and I came in periodically for family therapy sessions. I looked forward to these sessions because it was the one place that my family connected to each other in an honest way. It also gave me the opportunity to confront my father and express my anger toward him without retaliation.

I recall one of the sessions where Dr. Reiter brought in poetry by Kahlil Gibran. I still remember the lines, "Your children are not your children," and "The archer sees the mark upon the path of the infinite." Dr. Reiter asked each of us to choose either the bow, the arrow, or the archer and write about it in first person. My Dad wrote about being the archer and his being unsure that the arrow would hit its mark. My mom wrote about the bow and expressed her desire to stay strong and not crack. And I wrote about being an arrow, wondering if it would hit its target. I don't remember exactly what was said in that session, but I do remember my father crying and telling me he loved me. I also remember my mother crying and telling me she loved me. This encounter helped me to see the fact that my parents have their own insecurities, even my father.

How shocked I was to hear that my father was actually afraid of me when I yelled during confrontations at home. I knew there were times that my father tried to set limits with me, but he wasn't consistent. The truth was that I craved attention and discipline. I let my father know that I really needed structure and some parental control, and that his absence in my life was painful. He heard me. For a period of time, he started checking in with me every day to see how I was, and he tried to help me to structure my time more effectively. Truth be told, I was not always a willing participant. At times I was belligerent or avoidant. In therapy we contracted to spend father-son time together and to get to know each other. This worked out really well. Dad and I started to play golf, and we occasionally went out for lunch. I saw he was making an effort to be there for me.

Nevertheless, my problems did not disappear. My therapist had told me early on that there were medications that might help me with the mood swings. But why would I want to take some purple pill and become dependent on some chemical in my body? (For some reason, I didn't think of marijuana or alcohol in the same way). I resisted the idea of medication for five years. But at some point, I just hit bottom. I had failed three courses at the college I had transferred into and was afraid I would be kicked out again. I felt like I had fallen to the bottom of a great pit. And I needed help.

I had been avoiding my therapist for a couple of months, but now I asked for a family meeting at the therapist's office. Meanwhile, both of my parents and therapist believed that I was getting A's in college. I came clean in the session. I told them I had failed three courses. My father was stunned.

"I don't understand; I even saw your report card that said you got an A."

"I forged it."

No one said anything for a couple of minutes. Then my father said, "What do you want to do?" I replied that I didn't know what to do.

At this point my therapist intervened. "Mark, you've been in therapy now for six years. You've tried talk therapy, role-play, relaxation techniques, hypnotherapy, and family therapy. It's not working. There's only one thing you haven't tried—medication."

I had to admit that I had tried many different techniques to lower my anxiety and regulate my moods, and all had failed. With some trepidation, I made my way to a recommended psychiatrist. I understood that sometimes the medication had to be adjusted, and that it would take time.

The psychiatrist I went to charged $600 for the intake session. To add insult to injury, he sometimes fell asleep during the session and drooled onto his notebook! One time he asked me to help him with his paperwork and staple things for him during the session. Although his professional style left a lot to be desired, he played a critical role in finding the correct treatment for my mood disorder. After adjusting the dose, my moods became less erratic and my ability to concentrate improved. It was easier for me to get up in the morning and keep my commitments. I felt as though a great weight had been lifted from me.

> *Feelings of sorrow and guilt*
> *fly off my chest like birds*
> *I open up my self and shed*
> *the bouts of self-loathing*
> *every breath replacing the bad with God*
> *with the true self what my identity will truly behold*
> *no longer held back by the excess baggage of fear and doubt*
> *I feel lighter already*
> *The change of being, the transformations*
> *turn red of anger to the serenity of blue*
> *I am comfortable in my own shoes . . .*

This transformation was not easy, nor is it over. I still feel mood swings but I am not immobilized like before. I'm sorry I did not consider taking medication earlier; I would have spared myself so much emotional pain. I still need to work on being disciplined and responsible. My relationship with my mom and dad has improved, but it takes continuous effort.

I can't believe how much my life has changed within the last year. Several months ago I met a beautiful girl named Diana. I am learning what it is like to be in a real relationship. I have graduated from college—finally! It took three years longer than I expected, but I've got that diploma. I am leaving shortly for China to pursue my interest in international relations. I will need to return to school for a masters degree someday. But for now I want to see the world.

Notebook Entry—January 31, 2008

My true self has so many ambitions, held back in the past. I want to write. I want to create. There is so much in the world that I want to be a part of. It is my turn now.

I have hopes and dreams, and a great passion for life. I am going to continue to grow and give to my family and friends while I'm here. A generosity of self is what I would call it. I have held back this generosity; I have been unable to fully participate in the world. But not anymore. I can be so much to other people if I want to, and I do. The trappings of drugs and drink and conformity to others around me are no longer important.

"Tsunamis of sadness, fear and yearning / They crash over my huddling mortal soul" are the words of an adolescent overwhelmed with emotion. Mark writes of feeling trapped and alone. His mother's illness has made her more and more remote. His father is infrequently home. Emotionally, he feels abandoned. His anger is mixed with grief and loneliness. However, pen and paper are always accessible to him. The notebook is a love object, always present, attentive, and ready to receive his "secretions" of ink.

Mark's writing reflects several important therapeutic dimensions. First of all, he writes for catharsis and self-regulation of emotion. "My whole being only wishes to secrete feelings . . ." Secondly, he writes to organize and clarify thoughts and feelings. Thirdly, he writes for reflection, creating a safe space where he is not subject to others' opinions. Mark is trying to understand himself and problem-solve ("Who am I? / Where do I stand?") and his writing is filled with questions. Mark's notebook serves as his con-

fidante; he is writing to befriend and nurture himself, creating temporary "bandages for the holes in my soul." Mark also writes for self-discovery, wishing to comprehend his own connection to the universe. Last but not least, he writes for creativity and play. Most of the poems are written in the back of class, during periods of boredom.

Mark has a strong sense of the "imaginary audience."[3] In this phenomenon, first documented by Elkind (1967), the adolescent feels all eyes are upon him, evaluating his every move.[4] This feeling is exacerbated by Mark's social anxiety and depression. Mark feels as though he is under a microscope. However, when Mark reads his own writing, he has the opportunity to witness and view his own thoughts and feelings rather than be the object observed. This is satisfying because he experiences a sense of mastery and greater awareness while exercising his creativity.

When do Mark's problems begin? His mother's hospitalization seems to precipitate his downward spiral. Mark's mother returns home from the hospital in a wheelchair. That same year, Mark starts to feel paralyzed with social anxiety, particularly with members of the female gender. Years later he writes about watching his mother falling and collapsing and writes, "Oh, God, take me instead." Survivor guilt and Mark's powerful identification with his mother are contributing factors to his depression, but these factors alone are inadequate explanations for Mark's mood swings.

As with many people, Mark resisted going to a psychiatrist to be assessed. This is unfortunate, because his deep depressions could have been treated some years before. Although we are a modern and knowledgeable society, the stigma associated with going to a psychiatrist and taking medication still exists. As a result, many people do not seek the medical attention they need. Instead, the need to self-medicate led Mark to using marijuana and alcohol, which further obscured the primary problem. Talk therapy is not a panacea; it cannot correct an underlying chemical imbalance. However, talk therapy and writing therapy may provide support, remoralization, and catharsis. Together with medication, they may offer the best odds for complete recovery for those people who have mood disorders. It took Mark six years to accept the fact that he might need medication.

The difference in Mark's life was evident within several weeks. His words speak for themselves. "Feelings of sorrow and guilt/ fly off my chest like birds / I open up my self and shed the bouts of self-loathing." Mark is eager to participate in the world with what he calls "a generosity of self." In his last entry, he writes, "The trappings of drugs and drink and conformity to others around me are no longer important." Now twenty-four, Mark is finally free to become the man he wants to be. Self-acceptance is a necessary prerequisite for loving others. Mark's first romantic relationship is pivotal in his journey. In this relationship, he finds himself totally accepted and loved for who he is; he also is learning how his own ability to love can make a difference.

Mark's journey from adolescence to manhood was challenged by his family circumstances and his own biological predisposition. Individuation, the process of separating from one's family of origin and becoming one's own person, is undoubtedly one of the great transformations that occurs in the developmental life span of every human being. It takes each of us a lifetime to achieve.

Although in the process of writing this chapter Mark brought in notebook after notebook, he rarely brought his writing into therapy. Writing was the only place he could be 100 percent himself, without concern of his image in others' eyes. The notebook became the receptacle of his longings, his anxieties, his questions, and his reflections about life. The false persona that Mark erected to deal with the world could not help but fail ("I tried to be someone that I'm not.") The notebook was the one place undistorted by his need for social approval, a driving need to be accepted and respected. Even during the years that Mark hid behind a false persona, his true self was trying to emerge. The evidence is stashed away, hidden safely in his room. Mark's "notes from the back of the class" is a collection of lined notebook pages with almost illegible scribbles documenting an arduous "write of passage" into manhood.

~ 13 ~

The Journal That Was a Reservoir of Tears

Leah Tamar

Groucho Marx once said, "Aging is not a particularly interesting subject. Anyone can get old. All you have to do is live long enough."[1] However, aging may provide a unique opportunity for life review and reflection. Leah Schwartz is eighty years old and resides in an assisted living facility. Leah is deeply involved in the process of life review.

Life review is a universal and spontaneous event that naturally occurs during the developmental phase of growing older. Dr. Robert Butler, a gerontologist, suggested that it is the final opportunity for the individual to come to understand and resolve the conflicts of earlier life.[2] Both Butler and Dr. Erik Erikson have suggested that when conflicts are resolved, personality integration takes place and mortality is accepted.[3]

Leah has written sporadically throughout her life. Much writing has been done over the past eighteen years in therapy. At this time, because her eyes are weak, and writing is difficult, she dictates her thoughts and feelings to her poetry therapist, Dr. Reiter. Leah says, "I can't enter the real world, but I can still make my way onto the page."

This is Leah's story.

I'll be eighty this May. I live at the Ocean View Senior Home. I have plenty of time to think. So I think about my life. And all the business of living that remains an unfinished puzzle. I write because it helps me to put the pieces together. Sometimes writing helps me to remember the good things in life that I have experienced. At other times, I write about my regrets, my disappointments, and my angers. Writing gives me a place to put my tears. Tears are in more than half of my writings. I guess you could say my journal is a reservoir for me—a reservoir of tears.

Old age is a time for reflection. I still feel like a young girl inside and then I look in the mirror. What a shock! I find the fact that I am living in a building with elderly people extremely depressing. You ask, "Aren't you eighty?" Inside I feel as young as ever. I don't know what I'm doing in this place with so many old people.

Ode to the People of Ocean View Senior Living
The only time they focus is in the elevator
Their aim is to get downstairs to the dining room
They push, shove, and verbalize all the hostility they feel.
The humans have slipped to a lower level
The confusion in their minds turns to chaos . . .
I want to scream to the rooftops
the unfairness of it all
What can we do to give them back the security
of their younger years?
They cry out about the elevator on their way to dinner
But they are really crying
for a connection to Life
that is meaningful.

Where is meaning for me now? Where is my family? I have been divorced for the past twenty-five years. My two children, now in their forties, are out of the picture. Perhaps I see my daughter once every two or three years. My son rarely speaks to me. Aside from my therapist and the people who bring me my meals and shower me, there is little interaction with the world.

I am reminded of the words of the poet Edna St. Vincent Millay: "O world, I cannot get thee close enough." My closest friends are the characters of my soaps. The television is my most faithful companion. The comedies and tragedies of life continue to fascinate me. Perhaps at heart I am a frustrated dramatist, a would-be actress, a gypsy dancer that never got to perform. When did the ache in my heart first start? I wasn't always in mourning.

The Early Years

My childhood was joyous. I felt protected and loved. I was the apple of my father's eye, and even now, so many years later, I think about the time we spent together. Mama was often critical. Not much I did seemed to please her, but with my dad I could do no wrong. My happiest memories are of my dad dancing to music as I stood on his feet. He often took me to the movies, read to me, and taught me to appreciate music. When I was sick, I remember the gentleness of his hands laying cool cloths on my forehead. The sun rose and set with my father.

A Dance of Thanksgiving
There was a farm in Ferndale
My mother would take us across the road to this farm.
One day my father was wearing a blanket
Mom made for him—
out of pieces of baby blankets stitched together.
And my father climbed up on a large rock and began
*   to dance.*
I still see him on top of that rock
*   dancing.*
It was the equivalent of the Indian dance,
a dance of joy and celebration,
a dance giving thanks for all he had gotten.
We spent every summer upstate in a bungalow colony. These were

the most carefree, happy-go lucky days of my life. I will never forget those summers. I've written these poems to help me remember.

Summer in Ferndale

I carry warm milk in a turquoise bowl
straight from the cow to Mom.
My hand was so steady it didn't shake
once.
Then came the pleasure of drinking it
fresh from the mother cow—
My fondest memory of summer in Ferndale.

Happy Memories

I would skip along as we walked.
It started to shower.
I remember the sun on the leaves
as the rain fell.
Soon the rain stopped and
The sun came out strong once more.
We kept walking and singing.
That was my happiest day
totally filled with
the peacefulness of the country road.

I asked my father questions about God.
"Is he here?" "How do you know he's here?" "Is God in all the flowers?"
"Everywhere!" Dad said.
"How do you know?" I persisted.
Mama said, "All of this beauty is God's creation."
As far as Dad was concerned, God was everywhere.
Today I still wonder where God is.

As the first child of my parents, I had everyone's attention, especially my two sets of grandparents, my Bubbes and Zaydes, When my sister Linda was born, it was a rude awakening. My Zayde had just died, and in his place was this red-faced, crying imposter. In time, my little sister would drive me crazy with teasing; she knew exactly how to push my buttons. Linda grew up to be a judge, but even as a child she was bossy and always right. You would never guess that I was the older child. I have never gotten the best of her—except once and I wrote a poem about it.

Poem for My Sister

I hit her on the head with Webster's Unabridged Dictionary.
She made me do it.
That was glorious—the sound of that book hitting her head.
It was the only time I defeated her in seventy-six years!

I wanted more than anything to please Mama. She was a beautiful lady who was always busy cooking, cleaning, and gardening. When I think of Mama I think of her white gloves. She was seldom seen outside without those white gloves and a stylish hat. She wanted me to be a prim, proper young lady. Try as I might, I could not hold her attention—except when I did something wrong. Mama was judge, jury, and prosecutor. No matter what I did, it wasn't good enough.

I chose my dad as a role model. Once, when I was about six, I emulated him by going to the newsstand, waving my hand like Daddy did, and taking the newspaper home. Mama was aghast and insisted I take the newspaper back. She said I stole it. So I pretended to take the paper back, and, unbeknownst to her, threw it in the garbage when no one was looking.

I grew into a young woman who wanted to do her own thing. I was secretive because I knew Mama would not approve of my actions. I was young, rebellious, and insatiably curious about the opposite sex. I met many young men during my teens and into my twenties. I took a job as an accountant. Girlfriends were not so important to me. My parents would have been shocked if they knew of my liaisons. Fortunately, they never found out.

However, it was obvious that I was still single at the age of thirty.

Parental pressure and my own sense of "should" were the deciding factors in getting married. And Herbert seemed to fit the bill. He had a doctorate in anthropology. He was smart. He was a rebel in his own way, secretly storing away stolen library books, wheeling and dealing to make a buck and get the best deal. I thought I was in love. The first few years were happy ones.

I liked my new status as a married woman. I had two beautiful children, and I devoted myself to them. I went back to school to teach young children. I painted in my spare time and passionately created large canvases of oils in vibrant colors of cerulean blue, fuchsia, and vermilion.

THE FLOODGATES OPEN

I initially played the role of wife as I thought it should be played. I tried to please my husband. But at a certain point, a disquieting dissatisfaction set in. Did I delude myself? Perhaps Herbert was not the person I initially thought he was. The passage of the years and certain events would teach me that.

I had a healthy son and daughter when I found out that I was carrying twins. Carrying them was a time of great expectation and wonder. When they were stillborn, I was devastated. I never saw them. I never held them. I'm not sure I ever recovered from this loss. Even then, I wrote about my feelings.

> *It was a snowstorm.*
> *A blizzard was crying for them.*
> *The world was crying for them.*
> *The angels were crying for them.*
> *I didn't realize the extent of my devastation,*
> *still under anesthesia.*
> *The next day when it hit*
> *I couldn't accept it—*
> *I couldn't accept their death.*
> *Snow up to the knees,*

out of the hospital
I walked
in ice and snow I walked
inconsolable.

Later, when I came home, I learned that Herbert had the babies buried in Potters Field, with the poor and indigent. I think that is when I first knew that I would not stay married to him. His callousness was obvious. While he could be interesting and warm when he chose to be, he was often insensitive. I was horrified that he would allow his own children to be buried nameless in a graveyard for the poor. I would never forgive him for that.

Every parent who has lost a child wonders what he or she did to contribute to the loss. Did I do something to cause the babies' deaths? Was I using toxic paints when I created my art? Or did I take medicine that was harmful? I blamed myself. I did not touch my paints again. Something inside me closed up. I saw a counselor, who suggested I return to the classroom and devote my energy toward the children in my class. This action brought me some relief. I started teaching on the high-school level where I felt I could make a difference.

My unhappiness in my marriage persisted. At times Herbert seemed cold or indifferent. He spent much of the weekend away from me, visiting his friends. Was he having an affair? I was alone, except of course, when sexual services could be rendered. He was not interested in meeting my needs, only his own. I could have continued playing the role of the dutiful wife, but something in me snapped.

My sleep became erratic. My imagination, without the outlet of my painting, drew me to a world filled with shadow. I started to fast. I no longer held back my emotions. I let loose. I wept. I screamed. I ranted. Herbert had never seen me this way. He was mortified by my behavior and took me to doctor after doctor, convinced that I was either schizophrenic or a manic-depressive. I rearranged furniture in the middle of the night. Although I am only five feet tall, at this time I could move furniture that would take the strength of two men.

Deep down I knew that I wanted out of the marriage. In one of our screaming matches, Herbert asked me, "What do you want? Do you want a divorce?"

I screamed back, "Yes!" So why did it come as a shock when Herbert left?

This excerpt is from a much longer poem, written to capture the end of my twenty-five years of marriage. I remember driving in the car with Herbert after signing the divorce papers. He was crying, and I was unable to stop laughing. I wrote this poem after our divorce, when I realized how relieved I was that it was over.

> *The dam is ready to burst*
> *the waters trickle through*
> *I laughed*
> *no longer dammed*
> *till I cried*
> *no longer damned*

The years following the divorce were emotionally tumultuous. In spite of my mixed feelings toward Herbert, being single did not sit right with me. I felt "less than" without him. I needed to construct a new identity. I took workshops and tried to learn more about being on my own. I had no close friends. My children were grown and had flown the nest. My principal persuaded me to take an early retirement. It was a mistake. Without teaching I felt lost. There was a great vacuum in my life. Now the years of isolation began. The accumulation of all my losses weighed heavily. I sought intellectual and spiritual stimulation. One of the lectures I attended was about something I had never heard of— poetry therapy.

A Patchwork of Guilt

In my first session with Dr. Reiter, I wrote this poem:

The Phoenix of Spring
Guilt corrodes the key to my heart
It rusts the valves and tarnishes the vessel
Where the heart waits and waits.
I hear the crying of my heart
The flood of tears bursts forth . . .
The vessel cracks, needing mending . . .
It is broken . . . like my faith . . .
my dreams . . . my ideals . . .
my marriage . . . home . . . and family

Everything is broken!
Only my spirit survives . . .
Like the Phoenix
Out of black ash
Will come the green of life!
The green of spring
the yellow of daffodil
the red of rose!
Oh, Heart! There is so much beauty in this spring

There is no need to dwell on ash . . .
The phoenix of spring will flower once more!

You may ask, "How did the vessels of my heart corrode?" This is the part of the story that is difficult to share. Guilt played an important role in my life. Yes, a starring role. I had lost the twins. I had lost close contact with my children. I had lost my husband. Painting was also lost to me because I believed I had caused the miscarriage of the twins. I had woven an intricate patchwork of guilt and covered myself with this heavy blanket.

There were small transgressions, like the newspaper I stole and threw away despite Mama's insistence that I bring it back and confess. And then there was an early cross to bear—and I mean this literally. In kindergarten, one of the Christian children came up to me and punched me in the arm. "You killed our Lord, Jew."

I went home sobbing and although my mother said it was not true, I carried a burden of guilt. It became my mission not to upset anyone. Instead I would appease, acquiesce, submit, and do my best not to rock the boat. I lived with the terrible feeling that I had done something wrong and believed I deserved to be punished.

Perhaps it was this acquiescence, this easy submission that led to my worst transgression—an affair with a married man. I didn't mean for it to happen. But I didn't stop it either. How could a nice girl like me . . . ? During my last two years of marriage, it was like I was under a spell. I went through the motions of living like a robot. I was still married but felt very much alone. Herbert spent most of his free time with his friend, but not with me.

One day in the teacher's lounge, as I turned away from the file cabinet, my breasts accidentally brushed against a teacher standing behind me. And that's how the affair started. His reaction of delight led to a flirtation that was hard to resist. Chuck was a man well into his fifties who had a sense of humor and a strong sex drive. He found me sexy and entertaining. I made him feel young, and he made me feel like a woman.

We had one important thing in common. Our sexuality was defunct in our respective marriages. I no longer felt feminine in my marriage. And Chuck's masculinity was suffering; he was having difficulty performing sexually in his marriage ever since he started taking some high-blood-pressure medication. However, the grass is always greener on the other side. He never had trouble performing with me.

When I was with Chuck, I was funny and lighthearted. I had been buried in grief and depression for so long that I had lost those aspects of myself. Best of all, Chuck did not take me for granted. I found myself in an illicit relationship for almost a year. Until I decided it was over.

It was the mid-life affair of a menopausal woman. I kissed Chuck good-bye, and I walked away from my husband as well. I was self-sufficient financially and sexually too. I was tired of having to please and tired of acceptance that was conditional. I was fifty-five years old, and in many ways, going on eighteen. I was unsure of myself and trying to forge a new identity.

> I want to be me—
> I shift between needs and wants
> And lose sight of me.
> I want to be with others when I choose.
> I want to be free to leave when I choose.
> I want to have relationships with people with no strings
> Until I truly find me.
> I want things . . . I don't want things.
> I want people . . . I don't want people.
> I want order . . . I want chaos.
> I want the impossible.

I was an awkward late bloomer, finally on my own. It was a lonely life. But it was my life. Best of all, no one could tell me what to do. My sister and grown children tried. I was still sensitive to criticism and tended to vacillate in my decision-making, but I was becoming my own person.

The Golden Age
> I'm growing older.
> Stand, there in the dead of night.
> Sounds of silence penetrate deeply
> and crack the ice
> My tears rise to the surface
> I feel alive once more.

They say this is the "golden age." Actually, it might be more accurate to call it an age of rust, when no part of the body moves easily and the mind tends to vegetate.

247

Arthritis of the Mind

Burning joints . . .
 taut muscles . . .
  painful, unbending stiffness . . .
Unwillingness to change . . .
 to move forward
Tunnel vision and rigid point of view
Indicators of calcification of brain processes
 of atrophy of thought and deed . . .
  prejudice . . . emotional rigidity . . .
Will not get us through the pain in our minds.

I find being an older person is not only physically difficult, but emotionally challenging. Why? Let me explain.

Number One: Time is running out. It seems to be like a tape that speeds up as we near the end of the reel. Dr. Reiter tells me to "stay in the moment" and she asks me to focus on what I feel in the present. I dictate short poems that are like haikus. Here's one when I was feeling down:

> *I'm drowning in tears*
> *Depression overpowers me—*
> *Where is my cup of Jo?*

Here's one when I felt better:

> *The tears clear the veil*
> *I see again.*
> *The world is bright*

Number Two: People treat you like you're *non compos mentis*. Then you start to wonder if you are. I want to be treated like a person, not like a person who has lost her marbles.

I am not an Eskimo lady ready for an ice floe;
I don't want to be put out to pasture.
I don't want to drift off into the night.
I don't want anyone else telling me my time is up.
When I'm ready I'll close my eyes and drift off . . .

Number Three: Grown children devise ways to control your money. The struggle for power never ends. I've written many unsent letters to my children to clear myself of fury. I also wrote this short haiku for my son. It breaks the rules, just like he does:

He's tying my hands.
My wishes don't count.
He's doing it for my good—Ha! Ha!

Number Four: My requests are few and fairly simple. However, when you live in an assisted-living place, you depend on other people to get things for you. That can be a problem.

I don't ask for the sun and the moon—
just two bowls of oatmeal at breakfast,
yogurt or cottage cheese for lunch.
I'm not Boncha Schveig.
If you don't know who he is
read Sholom Aleichem.
By the way, where is my coffee or tea today?
Your water leaves much to be desired.
I want soy milk or soy milk—Take your choice!

Sometimes, probably because of the great amount of time I spend by myself, life becomes a blur. Occasionally, I go to sleep and lose track of time. The days are indistinguishable. My feelings swirl in my head and in my dreams, and it is easy to get lost in fog. But when I write, what I feel comes out in black and white. It is tangible and cannot be dismissed like a thought or feeling. And sometimes, I think, "Was it true?" The writing is a thread of evidence, a way to state the truth. It is important for me to hold on to the past—and let go of the past . . . to hold on to the present . . . and not to fear the future. Letting go and holding on and knowing when to do which—that's hard. My therapist tells me I need to make the most of my present life, despite its limitations. Easy to say, especially for a younger person.

I like to think that aging is a time of spiritual growth. Spirituality is the task of getting in touch with your own spirit and what makes you who you are. It is a time for making peace with those near and dear, even though I must confess that there are times I don't feel loving towards them. My sister still bosses me around. My grown children think they know what's best for me.

But every once in a while I experience a glimmer of hope. I now understand a truth that evaded me most of my life. My greatest regret is the fact that sometimes, because I wanted to gain approval, I undermined my own authority to please others. By doing so, I made it impossible to claim my own power, and find out who I am. I need to forgive myself for the betrayal of who I am—all the times I pleased others but in the process was not true to my own wants and needs. I need to forgive all the times my instinctive self has acted upon desire and later paid the price of guilt. I want a clean slate. I want to know that the good Lord will love me just the way I am.

> I want to be free of fear—
> The knowledge that I don't have to be perfect
> That I can make mistakes
> That I don't have to worry about others judging me
> That I don't have to make this last part of my life
> A statement to be judged in the hereafter.
> I want to know that God loves me.

The reservoir is full; the tears keep coming. Often a deep dissatisfaction wakens me in the middle of the night. Let me be honest—the world I am in is not what I want. I thought by now that I would have worked out the kinks in the puzzle of life. I hope I live a long time because I still have some things to work on. One of my paintings—that of a blue mountain top —hangs in my room.

> The climbing of mountains will be reserved for my dreams
> where I can do
> what I can't do in my waking hours . . .

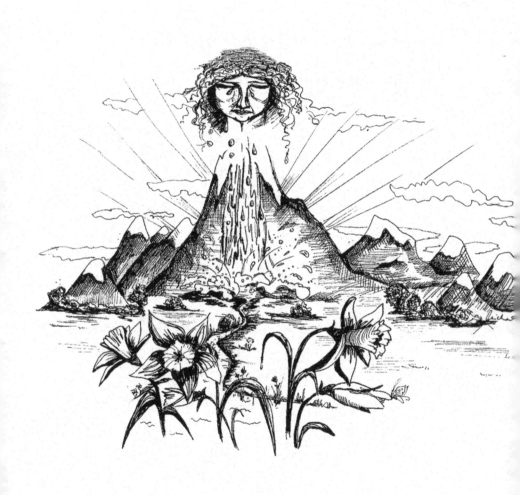

Leah is standing at the top of the mountain after climbing for many years. It is a unique vantage point from which to survey one's life. At eighty, Leah is still growing spiritually and psychologically. For some individuals, the hardest spiritual task of aging is standing before the Lord and accounting for one's deeds. Perhaps Leah's most difficult task is one of self-acceptance versus self-recrimination. "I need to forgive myself for the betrayal of who I am." The most powerful judge, jury, and prosecuter is not one's parent, husband, children, or even one's God; it is one's self.

Because writing transforms time, space, and matter, Leah is able to revisit her memories and expand those happy moments of childhood when she felt loved and protected. There is a tendency for older people either to inhabit the past with regrets or worry about the future. Through haiku and short poems, the poetry therapist encourages Leah to develop an awareness of staying in the present. "It is important for me to hold on to the past—and let go of the past . . . to hold on to the present . . . and not to fear the future. Letting go and holding on and knowing when to do which—that's hard." Such is the universal task of aging.

"The writing is a thread of evidence, a way to state the truth." The writing concretizes the memories and facilitates witnessing and reflection. For Leah, writing is empowering. Seeing her own truth in black and white is reaffirming, and in re-membering the fragmented memories, she can sense the greater wholeness of the life she has led. Leah's writing serves several purposes. She writes for clarification and organization; this is particularly important in the later years when memory may be limited and the mind sometimes lacks clarity. Leah uses the poems in the same way people use photo albums—to revisit the past and reflect upon it. She also writes in order to problem-solve, and to understand what she calls the "jigsaw puzzle" of her life.[4] Last but not least, Leah writes to express her feelings and this is often cathartic. Leah's poetry is filled with tears of sorrow, guilt, anger, and frustration.

Since Leah's moods swing from high to low, the goal of self-regulation is of primary importance. In "The Phoenix of Spring," the first poem she

writes in therapy, Leah rapidly switches her mood from despondency—
"Everything is broken!"—to the rapture of, "The green of spring / the yellow of daffodil / the red of rose. . ." This may indicate lability of mood or
the superimposing of hope over feelings of depression.

This first poem that Leah writes in therapy is like an emotional x-
ray, telling the clinician exactly what was happening through the poetic
device of metaphor: "Guilt corrodes the key to my heart / It rusts the
valves and tarnishes the vessel." These lines refer to Leah's psychological health. The lines also seem to intuit the subsequent deterioration of
her physical health from diabetes and arthritis. Corrosion and bitterness from multiple losses are laced with guilt and bitter self-recrimination. Had she caused the twins' death? The loss of her marriage? The
abandonment by her grown children? Was she in any way accountable
for the events in her life? In the next two decades we would explore
these questions.

Leah came from a highly protective environment with a critical mother
that she wanted to please. As a young woman she rebelled against others'
expectations and at the same time—paradoxically—tried to please others.
"My greatest regret is the fact that sometimes, because I wanted to gain
approval, I undermined my own authority to please others." When
approval rules us, many false masks are worn in order to appear beautiful
in the eye of the beholder. Leah was imprisoned by her own need to please
her mother and later her husband and children.

Some degree of psychological freedom has been restored to Leah
through the act of writing. She continues to work on saying what she
thinks and feels rather than what she "ought" to say. Writing provides
the safety that is sometimes lacking in face-to-face interaction. She is
learning to ask for what she wants: e.g. "I don't ask for the sun and the
moon—just two bowls of oatmeal at breakfast." In the last twenty-five
years she has exercised her right to take risks, delighting in occasionally
rocking the boat and making her voice heard.

It has been said that the record of each person's life, from infancy to
old age, is written in letters of tears. Crying serves an important pur-

pose, restoring emotional and biological equilibrium. Scientists who study the composition of emotional tears, have found hormones that build up to very high protein levels when the body withstands emotional stress. Tears are the natural solution for stress reduction and homeostasis.[5] Conversely, during the clinical state of depression, the body is in a shut-down state, and this self-healing process may not be easily accessed. Leah has discovered that tears and ink serve similar purposes—they are the tracings of the heart, leaving their tracks when the excesses of deep emotion overflow. Fortunately, there is a full reservoir of tears, and some of them are made of ink.

~ • ~

Conclusion

There is a Yiddish saying that God created humans because he loves a good story.[1] Poems are simply fragments of the larger life story. All of us live our stories, but not all of us are able to tell them. Some of us tell the story through art, music, dance, or theater. Sometimes, when the story is too new or raw with pain, it stays submerged in our hearts and minds; it may even live within the cells of our bodies. Sometimes, as in Maryellen's story of abuse and rape, the trauma is so deep, the story may stay silent for many years till a time of safety signals its release.

Humans are multi-storied. This fact means that when one story is destroyed, we create other stories. It also means that we have multiple stories and world views to choose from. Narrative therapy holds that our identities are shaped by the accounts of our lives; changing the story changes the life.[2] Because we organize our experience through story, there is a deep hunger to understand and share it with others.

Barry Lopez writes, "If stories come to you, care for them, and learn to give them away where they are needed. Sometimes a person needs a story more than food to stay alive."[3] Writing is a tool of psychological survival. It is a way of creating meaning in our lives, a way of reconciling our struggles and our triumphs, our helplessness and hopefulness in the labyrinth of emotional upheaval.

Sometimes a story is so powerful that instead of the person telling the story, the story tells the person! In other words, in Preston's story of war, his mind does not permit access to his memories of death and violence—till twenty-five years later. In Nadia's case, the story lives in her subconscious and informs her through dreams and nightmares. Poems and stories have a life of their own and sometimes the person is the last to know!

Following trauma, a story may defy articulation; it is jumbled, reflecting a thought process that needs time to organize its shape and meaning. If you are confronting a trauma experience, work with a professional ally; never stare a gorgon or a demon directly in the eye. When the terrain is dangerous, be sure to have a guide with you who knows the territory well.

Occasionally, the story becomes a scaffold, supporting one's identity. For example, in Susan's master narrative, her role as a doctor's wife is the organizing principle of her world. This storyline is hijacked when, instead of being "the doctor's wife," she becomes a prisoner's wife. An identity crisis is inevitable. However, stories are chameleons. In time, they will transform. If we visit Susan today, we may find she has gone beyond her master narrative into an alternative one. In all likelihood, she is a different woman, in a new career, perhaps even in a new relationship. If we hold on to the same story for dear life, it becomes like stale bread. It is inedible and cannot nurture you or anyone else. Don't cry—let it go. Make room in your life for something new and alive.

"You can't order a poem like a taco," as Naomi Shihab Nye has written.[4] It takes time for a story to grow inside one's life, and make its way into the external world. Most of the stories and poems in this book slept for five, ten, twenty or more years in a journal before they were brought into the light. When we live too close to the story, we may not be able to see it or sense the whole of it. Stories cannot be rushed. Like fruit, they ripen in their own best season.

Nor can the story be hunted like prey. It is not a possession to be guarded zealously; the ego and its defenses tend to get in the way of the story. Ambivalent emotions may also constrict the writer. For example, one story about a father's abuse could not be submitted. The father was on his deathbed, and the son, overwhelmed with guilt and ambivalent feelings of loss, could not malign his dying father. Stories of integrity require absolute fidelity. Loyalty to others may muddy the storyline. "How will my children feel if they read my story?" "What would my husband say if he knew about the affair?" "What will my parents say if they learn about the abortion?" Three writers chose to use alias names to protect their privacy. The issue of safety is a prerequisite to self-disclosure. We cannot stay completely true to our story if we are censoring it to protect others. On the other hand, sometimes we may censor ourselves for purposes of self-protection. When insights of the heart and mind are painful, they are not always welcomed into the light of consciousness.

Could you sense when there was something the writer was holding back? Omissions speak volumes. Were you able to read between the lines? As readers, we usually fill in the blanks with our imagination. However, when the author chooses to conceal rather than reveal, we distance ourselves from the story or perhaps more accurately, the story distances itself from us. It may be argued that a story is never totally complete because it is always a fragment of larger experience, always limited by the vantage point of the writer. The best that we can do is find words that ring with integrity to articulate our thoughts and feelings at any given moment in time. And when we are successful, there is a deep and glorious satisfaction.

Every time a person writes, it is an attempt to understand where one has been, and where one is going. The writing serves as an invaluable compass in understanding the geography of one's life. A *New York Times* article (May 22, 2007) states, "Mental resilience relies in part on . . . this kind of autobiographical storytelling, moment to moment, when navigating life's stings and sorrows."[5] Despite the disorder and chaos that often comes with change, creative coping holds seeds for a new existence. Resilience or hardiness is the ability to adapt to new circumstances when life presents the unpredictable. According to psychologist Salvatore R. Maddi, hardiness or resilience comes through commitment, control, and challenge.[6] Not surprisingly, the creative process encompasses these three elements.

It is a creative act of courage to tell the story and write the poem, to encounter one's griefs, angers, and shame, and to choose a creative channel to intentionally funnel one's emotions. Some authors charted their journeys on their own. Others enlisted the aid of a therapist as guide. *All of the authors chose creative coping.* They finished the poem and told the story rather than react with the more usual stress responses (fight, flight, or freeze). As a result, they were able to minimize disorientation, numbness, and emotional discomfort. All of the writers harnessed the restorative capacity of writing to identify, organize, contain, and release their stories.

The contributors have shared their writings in the hopes that you will be inspired and strengthened by their words. In the last section of this book, there are resources for the writer who lives within you. Perhaps you will be brave enough to pick up that pen and write your own story.

~ • ~

End Notes

INTRODUCTION

1. H. Stefan Bracha et al., "Does Fight or Flight Need Updating?" *Psychosomatics* 45 no. 5 (2004) 448-449, www.psy.psychiatryonline.org/cgi/content/full/45/5/448 (accessed January 26, 2009). If you are interested in further reading on stress, see the landmark classic: Hans Selye, *The Stress of Life* (New York: McGraw-Hill, 1978). For a more recent publication, see Richard S. Lazarus, *Stress and Emotion: A New Synthesis* (New York: Springer Publishing Co., 2006).
2. Friedrich Nietszche, *Thus Spoke Zarathustra* (New York: Penguin Books, 1978). The quote originally appeared in Nietszche's book *Twilight of the Idols* in 1888.
3. Jane Hope, *The Secret Language of the Soul* (San Francisco, CA: Chronicle Books, 1997), 111.
4. Edward Hirsch, *The Demon and the Angel: Searching for the Source of Artistic Inspiration* (New York: Harcourt, Inc., 2002), xii-xiii.
5. The concept of duende is best explained in Garcia Lorca's lecture, "Play and Theory of the Duende," first given in Buenos Aires in 1933, and available online: http://www.tonykline.co.uk/PITBR/ Spanish/LorcaDuende.htm.

WRITING AWAY THE DEMONS

6. Caryn Mirriam-Goldberg, *The Power of Words* (Keene, New Hampshire: Transformative Language Arts Press, 2007), 12.
7. *The National Association for Poetry Therapy* (NAPT Brochure). Pembroke Pines, Florida: NAPT, c. 1995. According to the NAPT brochure, "Poetry therapy, journal therapy and bibliotherapy are terms used synonymously to describe the intentional use of the written or spoken word by a trained biblio/poetry/journal therapist." For more information about poetry therapy, see www.poetrytherapy.org and www.nfbpt. com for the *National Federation for Biblio/Poetry Therapy*. Poetry Therapy, Bibliotherapy, and Journaling evolved from different sources: "Poetry Therapy" harkens back to ancient times when the Greeks worshipped Apollo, the god of medicine as well as poetry. The field of poetry therapy was officially established in the twentieth century with the publication of psychiatrist Jack J. Leedy's book: *Poetry Therapy* and the subsequent founding of the *Association for Poetry Therapy* (1969), converted into the *National Association for Poetry Therapy* (1982). "Bibliotherapy," a form of supportive psychotherapy, was first employed by librarians during and following World War I, in which carefully selected reading materials were prescribed to assist veterans in solving personal problems. Bibliotherapy evolved out of library science. Rhea Rubin, *Bibliotherapy Sourcebook* (Phoenix, AZ: Oryx Press, 1978). "Journaling," self-guided writing for personal growth and healing, became a popular art form in the last century due to four trained psychotherapists: Carl Jung, Marion Milner, Ira Progroff and Anais Nin. For more information, see Tristine Rainer, *The New Diary* (Los Angeles: J.P. Tarcher, 1978), 21.
8. James W. Pennebaker, *Opening Up: The Healing Power of Confiding in Others* (New York: Morrow, 1990).
9. Stephen Lepore, and Joshua Smyth, eds., *The Writing Cure: How Expressive Writing Promotes Health and Emotional Well-Being* (Washington, D.C.: American Psychological Association, 2002).
10. Kathleen Adams, *Journal to the Self: Twenty-Two Paths to Personal Growth* (New York: Warner Books, 1990).

11. Stephen Quirk, *Who Were the Pharoahs?: A History of Their Names with a List of Cartouches* (London, U.K.: Thames and Hudson, 1996).

12. Benjamin Mazar, "Jerusalem in the Biblical Period" in Yigael Yadin, ed., *Jerusalem Revealed* (Jerusalem: Israel Exploration Society, 1976).

13. Helen Keller, Roger Shattuck, Dorothy Hermann, and Anne Sullivan, *The Story of My Life: The Restored Classic, Complete and Unabridged, Centennial Edition* (New York: W.W. Norton & Co., 2003). The naming of water is also powerfully portrayed in *The Miracle Worker*, the film that won Patty Duke and Ann Bancroft Oscars in 1962.

14. Jeanne Achterberg, and Barbara Dossey, *Rituals of Healing; Using Imagery for Health and Wellness* (New York: Bantam Books, 1994).

15. Kate Thompson, "Journal Writing as a Therapeutic Tool" in Gillie Bolton, Stephanie Howlett, Colin Lago and Jeannie K Wright, eds., *Writing Cures: An Introductory Handbook of Writing in Counselling and Therapy* (New York: Brunner-Routledge, 2004), 72.

16. Ronald Pies, "The Poet and the Therapist," in the *Journal of Poetry Therapy, the Interdisciplinary Journal of Practice, Theory, Research and Education*, 22 (1988): 84-88.

17. imallowed.com/five_freedoms.html (accessed March 1, 2009). To learn more about Virginia Satir's work, see these classics: Virginia Satir, *Self-Esteem* (Berkeley, CA: Celestial Arts, 2001), and Virginia Satir, *The New Peoplemaking* (Palo Alto, CA: Science and Behavior Books, 1988).

18. Tristine Rainer, *The New Diary* (Los Angeles, CA.: J.P. Tarcher, 1978), 69.

19. Walt Whitman, *Leaves of Grass*; New York Public Library Collector's Edition (Garden City, NY: Doubleday & Co., Inc., 1926), 76.

20. Jack J. Leedy and Sherry Reiter, "Poetry in Drama Therapy," in Gertrud Schattner and Richard Courtney, eds., *Drama in Therapy*, Volume II, Adults (NY: Drama Book Specialists, 1981), 224.

21. Morris Morrison, *Poetry as Therapy* (New York: Human Sciences Press, 1987), 23.

22. Jean Cocteau, *Opium: The Diary of a Cure* (London, Peter Owen, 1930), 139.

23. Geraldine Pinch, *Magic in Ancient Egypt* (London: British Museum Press, 1994). For a complete history of poetry therapy, download the National Federation for Biblio/Poetry Therapy Training Guide at www.nfbpt.com.

24. Frank Wilson, *The Hand: How Its Use Shapes the Brain, Language and Human Culture* (NY: Vintage Books, 1999).

25. Daniel Goleman, *Emotional Intelligence* (NY: Bantam Books, 1994), 294.

26. Hannah Arendt, *The Human Condition* (Chicago: IL.: University of Chicago Press, 1958), 175. This quote originally appeared in a telephone interview published in *The New York Times Book Review*, November 3, 1957 as follows: "One of my friends said about me that I think all sorrows can be borne if you put them into a story or tell a story about them, and perhaps this is not entirely untrue."

27. Jack J. Leedy and Sherry Reiter, "The Uses of Poetry in Drama Therapy," in Gertrud Schattner and Richard Courtney, eds., *Drama in Therapy*, Volume II (New York: Drama Book Specialists, 1981), 224.

28. Ron Padgett, *The Teachers and Writers Handbook of Poetic Forms* (NY: Teachers & Writers Collaborative, 2000), 119.

29. Silvano Arieti, *Creativity: The Magic Synthesis* (New York: Basic Books, 1976), 54-55.

30. Gary Snyder, *The Practice of the Wild* (Berkeley, CA: North Point, 1990).

31. Mary Caroline Richards, *Centering: In Pottery, Poetry and the Person* (Middletown, CT: Wesleyan University Press, 1962), 18.

32. Ibid, 18.

33. Hans R. Scholer, "The Potential of Stem Cells: An Inventory" in Nikolaus Knoepffler, Dagmar Schipanski, and Stefan Lorenz Sorgner, eds. *Humanbiotechnology As Social Change* (Burlington, VT: Ashgate Publishing, 2007).

34. Wallace Bacon, *The Art of Interpretation* (New York: Holt, Rinehart and Winston, Inc., 1966).

35. Melissa Reed, "Shakespeare's Poetics of Play-Making and Therapeutic Action," *Journal for Poetry Therapy, The Interdisciplinary Journal of Practice, Theory, Research and Education*, Volume 14, Number 1, (Fall 2000): 25.

36. Christina Baldwin, *One-to-one: Self-Understanding through Journal Writing* (New York: A. Evans & Co., 1977), 9.

37. Ibid., 15.

38. Jeanne Achterberg and Barbara Dossey, *Rituals of Healing; Using Imagery for Health and Wellness* (New York: Bantam Books, 1994), 9.

CHAPTER 1

1. Patrick Riley, ed., *The Cambridge Companion to Rousseau* (Cambridge, MA: Cambridge University Press, 2001).

2. Hortense Calisher, "Sunbeams," *The Sun*, Issue 332 (August 2003): 1.

3. Verse: from Latin versus "a turn of the plow, a furrow, a line of writing," from vertere 'to turn' hacker. 2008. In *Merriam-Webster Online Dictionary*, http://www.merriam-webster.com/dictionary/hacker.

4. Seamus Heaney and Sam Leith, "'Dig It Out!'"—Seamus Heaney Talks to Sam Leith about Poetry," *Kitabkhana*, Saturday, May 27, 2006. blogspot.com/2006/05/dig-it-out-seamus.heaney (accessed September 7, 2008).

5. Joan Acocella, "On the Contrary: A New Look at the Work of H.L. Mencken," *The New Yorker*, 17 July, 2008.

6. Melody Beattie, *Co-Dependent No More: How to Stop Controlling Others and Start Taking Care of Yourself* (Center City, MN: Hazelden, 1992). In addition to Beattie's classic, see Pia Mellody, Andrea Wells Milner and J. Keith Miller, *Facing Co-Dependence: What It is, Where It comes From, How It Sabotages Our Lives* (New York: Harper & Row, 1989); Janae B. Weinhold, Barry K. Weinhold, and John Bradshaw, *Breaking Free of Co-dependency* (Novato, CA: New World Library, 2008).

CHAPTER 2

1. For a greater understanding of traumatic experience, read Jonathan Shay, *Achilles in Vietnam: Combat Trauma and the Undoing of Character* (New York: Simon & Schuster, 1995); Edward Tick, *War and the Soul; Healing Our Nation's Veterans from Post-Traumatic Stress Disorder* (Wheaton, IL: Quest Books, 2005); Peter Levine, *Healing Trauma: The Innate Capacity to*

Transform Overwhelming Experience (Berkeley, CA: North Atlantic Books, 2008).

2. Eric Rudder Eddison, *The Worm Ouroboros* (New York: E.P. Dutton, 1952). The fascinating history of the ouroboros is more recently available online or in print. See Eric Rucker Eddison and Keith Henderson, *The Worm Ouroboros* (New York: BiblioBazaar, 2008).

3. Dr. Jack J. Leedy, "Poetry Therapy for Drug Abusers," *The American Journal of Social Psychiatry VII*, 2, (Spring 1987): 108. The author has borrowed the concept of converting blood to ink from Dr. Jack Leedy, who used the term in a different way, referring to depressed and suicidal patients. He suggested that when his suicidal patients donate a pint of blood, often their suicidal trends are alleviated; the poem symbolically represents an organ or pint of blood, and is thereby helpful therapeutically. "Writing a poem is like converting blood to ink"(108). Dr. Leedy was fond of saying that in the Supreme Court of the mind, the internal debates of a depressed person could result in a five to four decision: five factors that make life intolerable vs. four encouraging the patient to go on living. Writing converts one vote from death to life.

CHAPTER 3

1. Friedrich Nietszche, *Thus Spoke Zarathustra* (New York: Penguin Books, 1978). (Originally published in 1881).

2. http:/www.breastcancer.org (accessed January 19, 2009).

3. htttp//www.ascendfoundation.org/facts_06.html from American Cancer Society To learn more about breast cancer, see the following sites: www.breastcancer.org, www.oncolink.com, www.cancer.org, and www.cancercenter.com For helpful books about cancer, see Lori Hope, *Help Me Live: Twenty Things People With Cancer Want You to Know* (Berkeley, CA: Celestial Arts, 2005); Susan Love, M.D., *Dr. Susan Love's Breast Book: 4th Edition* (New York: Da Capo Press, 2005).

4. The concrete poem is a poetic form, in which the words dramatize their meaning by the way they look and how the words are spaced on the page. For more information, see Ron Padgett, *The Teachers and Writers*

Handbook of Poetic Forms (New York: Teachers & Writers Collaborative, 2000).

5. There are many fine examples of women writing their way through cancer, as exemplified in Sharon Bray, *When Words Heal: Writing through Cancer* (Berkeley, CA: Frog Ltd., 2006); Myra Schneider, *Writing My Way through Cancer* (London, U.K.: Jessica Kingsley Publishers, 2003).

CHAPTER 4

1. Theresa Cole, *Splintered Emotions: Aftermath of Child Abuse* (Indianapolis, IN: Oberpark Publishing, 2006). According to Theresa Cole, results of abuse include: self-doubt, low self esteem, confusion, apathy, depression, suspicion, hypervigilance, fear, anger, rage, sadness, mistrust, nightmares, and later in life frequently addiction, alcoholism, domestic violence, and more child abuse. For an in-depth look at the results of child abuse, see Lisa Aronson Fontes, *Child Abuse and Culture: Working with Diverse Families* (London: The Guilford Press, 2008). Teens and adults who have been abused may benefit from reading Patricia Evans, *The Verbally Abusive Relationship: How to Recognize It and How to Respond* (Cincinnati, Ohio: Adams Media, 2003).

2. Pat Conroy and Suzanne Williamson Pollack, *The Pat Conroy Cookbook: Recipes of My Life* (New York: John Wiley, 2004).

3. www.healingplace.info/resources/virginia_satir/
To learn more about Virginia Satir's work, see Virginia Satir, *Self-Esteem* (Berkeley, CA: Celestial Arts, 2001). Also see Virginia Satir, *The New Peoplemaking* (Palo Alto, CA: Science and Behavior Books, 1988).

4. Suniya Luthar, *Resilience and Vulnerability: Adaptation in the Context of Childhood Adversities* (Cambridge, U.K.: Cambridge University Press, 2003). The subject of why some children who have faced major stressors do not develop severe psychological symptoms has fascinated mental health professionals for many years. Stressors appear to have a cumulative effect, but having at least one healthy and loving relationship makes a decisive difference. For more information on resilience, see social worker Nan Henderson's website featuring "The Resilience Wheel." To take a

quiz to discover if conditions in your life are fostering resiliency, see www.resiliency.com/htm/resiliencyquiz.htm.

CHAPTER 5

1. Stephen Mitchell, ed., *The Selected Poetry of Rainer Maria* (New York: Vintage International, 1989). This famous passage is the first of the Duino Elegies by Rainer Maria Rilke:

   Who if I cried out would hear me among the angels' hierarchies
   and even if one of them pressed me suddenly against his heart:
   I would be consumed in that overwhelming existence.

2. For a greater understanding of surviving sexual abuse and trauma, see Ellen Bass and Laura Davis, *The Courage to Heal: A Guide to Survivors of Sexual Abuse*, 4th Edition (New York: Collins Living Publishers, 2008); Judith Lewis Herman, *Father-Daughter Incest* (Cambridge, MA: Harvard University Press, 2000).

3. The essential feature of dissociative disorders is a disruption in the usually integrated functions of consciousness, memory, identity or perception. For specifics, see *Diagnostic Statistical Manual IV T-R* (Text Revision) (Arlington, VA: American Psychiatric Association, 2000).

4. Edward Hirsch, *The Demon and the Angel: Searching for the Source of Artistic Inspiration* (New York: Harcourt, Inc., 2002).

5. Susan C. Feldman, David Read Johnson & Marilyn Ollayos, "The Use of Writing in the Treatment of Post-Traumatic Stress Disorders" in John F. Sommer and Mary Beth Williams, eds. *The Handbook of Post-Traumatic Therapy* (Westport, Connecticut: Greenwood Publishing 1994), 366-385.

CHAPTER 6

1. booksafe.com/nautical-knowhow/marktwain.htm
   Samuel Clemens worked as a steamboat captain. "Mark Twain" was the frequent call on the river, signifying that the water was twelve feet deep and considered safe water. Clemens took on the name Mark Twain to keep the memories of his happy days on the river with him.

2. Eli Greifer, *Principles of Poetry Therapy* (New York: Poetry Therapy Center,

1963).

3. Ibid., 2. Greifer's words are eloquent: "We have here no less than a psychograft-by-memorization in the inmost reaches of the brain, where the soul can allow the soul-stuff of stalwart poet-prophets to "take" and to become one with the spirit of the patient. Here is insight. Here is introjection. Here is ennoblement of the spirit of man . . . by blood transfusing the personality with the greatest insights of all the greatest-souled poets of all ages . . . The hypnotism of beautiful figures of speech, the melody of rhythm and meter and assonance . . . painted scenes . . . dramatic episodes, love's pervasiveness—all are consecrated by the master poets to gently enter and transfuse the ailing subconscious, the abraded and suffering personality."

CHAPTER 7

1. The author describes her anger, sense of betrayal, and a sadness that turns into a melancholy following the abortion that was to last for the next two decades. The poem "Cyclone" captures the sense of violent devastation and loss of control she experienced. For a greater understanding of possible consequences of abortion, see Barbara Horak, *Real Life Abortion Stories: The Hurting and the Healing* (Topeka, KS: Strive for the Best Publishing, 2007).

2. Mourning is incomplete because it is forbidden. Family and society do not acknowledge the pregnancy, much less the abortion. For a greater understanding of complicated mourning, see Theresa Rando, *Treatment of Complicated Mourning* (Champagne, IL: Research Press, 1993). Specific to mourning in abortion, see David C. Reardon, and Theresa Burke, *Forbidden Grief: The Unspoken Pain of Abortion* (San Francisco, CA: Acorn Books, 2007).

3. Robert Campbell, "God, Man, and Whale." *New York Times*, July 20, 2008. Kunitz believed poems exist before you know them: "Even before it is ready to change into language, a poem may begin to assert its buried life in the mind with wordless surges of rhythm and counter rhythm."

4. Jack J. Leedy and Sherry Reiter, "Poetry in Drama Therapy," in Gertrud

Schattner and Richard Courtney, eds., *Drama in Therapy*, Volume II, Adults (NY: Drama Book Specialists, 1981), 224.

CHAPTER 8

1. According to the National Institute on Aging, there are 4.5 million people in the United States with Alzheimers. To know more about this disease, see U.S. National Institutes of Health, National Institute on Aging www.nia.nih.gov/alzheimers, and Alzheimer's Association at www.alz.org.

2. In the classic Greek mythological tale, Sisyphus uses chains to lock up Death, so that no mortal can die. There are many variations of this tale, and in one of them, Sisyphus steals Death's pen so he cannot write in the Book of Death. To read about Sisyphus and other myths, see Liz Greene and Juliet Sharman-Burke, *The Mythic Journey: The Meaning of Myth as a Guide for Life* (New York: Simon & Schuster, 2000).

3. Alzheimer's results in complicated grief because the family is subjected to a long, extended mourning as the person that they knew ceases to exist, but their physical presence continues. For more information, see Elizabeth Forsythe, *Alzheimer's Disease: The Long Bereavement* (London, U.K.: Faber & Faber, 1990).

4. Words are the first auditory connection between infant and mother. Even though they may not be understood, the sound of the human voice is comforting and familiar because it is heard in utero. The author is trying to use words to connect, even though at times his mother does not recognize him and responsiveness is limited. It is a challenge to connect and honor such a person. See Nancy Pearce, *Inside Alzheimer's: How to Hear and Honor Connecting with a Person Who Has Dementia* (Taylors, S.C.: Forasson Press, 2007).

5. Liz Greene and Juliet Sharman-Burke, *The Mythic Journey: The Meaning of Myth as a Guide for Life* (New York: Simon and Schuster, 2000). In the myth, Hades promised Sisyphus that if he ever succeeded in pushing the rock over the top and to the other side, his punishment would end. Although Sisyphus heaved the boulder to the edge of the slope, the rock always tricked him, slipping out of his grasp and chasing him down the

hill. Such an act of utter frustration and pointless repetition is often referred to as a Sisyphian task or challenge.

CHAPTER 9

1. *Domestic Violence First Quarter Fact Sheet Year 2008.*
   www.nyc.gov/html/ocdv/downloads/pdf/Fact Sheet 2008_1ˢᵗ Q.pdf
   Domestic Violence U.S. Resources www.vachss.com/help_text/domestic_violence_us.html
   For more information on domestic violence, see *The Domestic Violence Awareness Handbook,* published by the Safety, Health, Employee and Welfare Division, is available online: www.usda.gov/da/shmd/aware.htm; Lisa A. Goodman, Deborah Epstein, and Judith L. Herman, *Listening to Battered Women: A Survivor-centered Approach to Advocacy, Mental Health and Justice* (Psychology of Women) (Washington, D.C.: American Psychological Association, 2007); Judith Lewis Herman, *Trauma and Recovery: The Aftermath of Violence from Domestic Violence to Political Terror* (New York: Basic Books, 1997).
2. http://lynneforrest.com/html/the_faces_of_victim.html (accessed November 8, 2008).
3. www.imallowed.com/five_freedoms.html (accessed March 1, 2009).
4. Stephen Karpman, "Fairy Tales and Script Drama Analysis," *Transactional Analysis Bulletin,* 1968 7(26), 39-43. The Drama Triangle is a high energy blame game involving rescue and drama. The triangle has been written up in many Transactional Analysis books including texts by Eric Berne, Muriel James, Ianne Stewart and Vann Joines. Games, according to Karpman, are played at a first, second or third degree intensity. Barbara and Lafayette were playing the game at Level 3. For more information, check the ITAA-net.org website or the many articles online at www.karpmandramatriangle.com.

CHAPTER 10

1. To learn more about the experience of wives and families of persons serving time in prison, see Laura T. Fishman, *Women at the Wall: A Study of*

Prisoners' Wives Doing Time on the Outside (New York: State University of New York, 1990); Dave J Hardwick, *Serving the Second Sentence; Survival Guide for Wives and Families of Prisoners* (London, UK: Prepar, Ltd., 1986).

Chapter 11

1. For information on Multiple Sclerosis, see Barbara Giesser, Rosalind Kalb, Nancy Holland, and David Lander, *Multiple Sclerosis for Dummies* (Hoboken, N.J: For Dummies, 2007). For understanding the psychological component of MS, see Allison Shadday and Stanley Cohan, *MS and Your Feelings: Handling the Ups and Downs of MS* (Alameda, CA: Hunter House, 2006). For online information, see www.webmd.com/multiple-sclerosis/default.htm

2. For more information on disability from a psychological and philosophical vantage point, see Lennard Davis, *The Disability Studies Reader*, 2nd Ed. (London: Routledge, 2006); Lennard Davis and Michael Berube, *Bending Over Backwards: On Disability and the Body* (New York: NYU Press, 2002).

3. Here Nancy is choosing to be a disabled hero, one of the topics explored in Susan Wendell, *The Rejected Body: Feminist Philosophical Reflections on Disability* (Charlotte, NC: Routledge, 1996).

4. The person who is disabled and isolated from society is at risk for becoming alienated and depressed. Carol Gill, a disabled psychologist, suggests an alternative. Carol Gill, "A Psychological View of Disability Culture," *Disability Studies Quarterly* (Fall 1995). Article may be viewed online at: www.independentliving.org/docs3/gill1995.html

CHAPTER 12

1. John Keats, *Endymion*, 1818.

2. Robert Feldman, *Development Across the Life Span* (Upper Saddle River, NJ: Prentice Hall, 2003).

3. One in eight teens may be suffering from depression, and it is thought that only thirty percent of the teens suffering from emotional turmoil are receiving treatment. Depression and mood disorders are fairly common in the

United States, with anti-depressants being more prescribed than any other drug. To learn more, see Peter C. Whybrow, *A Mood Apart: The Thinker's Guide to Emotion and Its Disorder* (New York: Harper, 1998); Bev Cobain, Peter S. Jensen, and Elizabeth Verdick, *When Nothing Matters Anymore; A Survivor's Guide for Depression* (Minneapolis, MN: Free Spirit Publishing, 2007). Specifically to address teen depression, see Faye Zucker, and Joan E. Huebl, *Teens Find Light at the End of the Tunnel* (Danbury, CT: Franklin Watts, 2007).

4. David Elkind, "Egocentrism in Adolescence," *Child Development*, 38 (1967): 1025-1034. Imaginary audience is an adolescent's egocentric belief that his or her own behavior is a primary focus of others' attentions and concerns; it may result in self-consciousness and the adolescent may create imaginative scenarios about what others are thinking about them. David Elkind was the first to write about it in 1967.

Chapter 13

1. The quote is attributed to Groucho Marx, exact source unknown.
2. Robert N. Butler, "The Life Review: An Unrecognized Bonanza," *International Journal of Aging and Human Development* 12 (1980): pp. 35-38. Also see Robert N. Butler, "The Life Review: An Interpretation of Reminiscence in the Aged," *Psychiatry* 26 (1963): 65-75.
3. Erik Erikson, *The Life Cycle Completed* (New York: W.W. Norton, 1982). Also see: Erik Erikson, "Identity and the Life Cycle: Selected Papers," *Psychological Issues* 1 (1959): 50-100.
4. Putting the pieces together to understand one's life as a whole is the goal. It has been most poignantly expressed by May Sarton through a fictitious elderly character: "I am keeping a journal. I call it *The Book of the Dead*. By the time I finish it I shall be dead. I want to be ready, to have gathered everything together and sorted it out, as if I were preparing for a great final journey. I intend to make myself whole here in this Hell. It is the thing that is set before me to do. So, in a way, this path inward and back into the past is like a map, the map of my world. If I can draw it accurately, I shall know where I am." May Sarton, *As We Are Now* (New York: W.W.

Norton & Co., 1992).

5. William Frey, Crying: *The Mystery of Tears* (Minneapolis, MN: Winston Press, 1977). Also see Gregg Levoy, "The Tears That Speak," *Psychology Today* (July-August, 1988).

CONCLUSION

1. Steve Zeitlin, *Because God Loves Stories* (New York: Simon and Schuster, 1997). Some attribute this quote to Reb Nachman of Bratzlav, but its exact source is not known.

2. For more information on narrative therapy, see: Gerald Monk, John Winslade, Kathie Crocket, and David Epston, *Narrative Therapy in Practice: The Archaeology of Hope* (Hoboken, NJ: Jossey Bass; David Epston and Michael White, *Narrative Means to Therapeutic Ends* (New York: W.W. Norton, 1990).

3. Barry Lopez, *Crow and Weasel* (New York: Farrar, Straus, and Giroux, 1998), 45.

4. Naomi Shihab Nye, *The Red Suitcase* (Brockport, New York: BOA Editions, 1994).

5. Benedict Carey, "'This Is Your Life—(And How You Can Tell It),'" *New York Times*, May 22, 2007, Health/Mental Health & Behavior.

6. Salvatore R. Maddi, "Hardiness: An Operationalization of Existential Courage," *Journal of Humanistic Psychology* 44, no.3 (July 2004): 279-298.

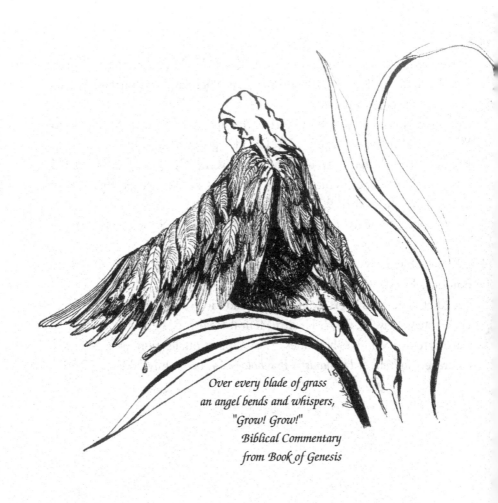

Over every blade of grass
an angel bends and whispers,
"Grow! Grow!"
Biblical Commentary
from Book of Genesis

~ • ~

Recommended Reading for the Writer in You

Adams, Kathleen. *Journal to the Self: Twenty-Two Paths to Personal Growth.* NY: Warner, 1990.

Adams. Kathleen. *The Way of the Journal: A Journal Therapy Workbook for Healing.* Baltimore, MD: The Sidran Institute Press, 1998.

Addonizio, Kim and Dorianne Laux. *The Poet's Companion: A Guide to the Pleasures of Writing Poetry.* NY: W.W. Norton & Co., 1997.

Addonizio, Kim. *Ordinary Genius: A Guide for the Poet Living Within.* NY: WW Norton & Co., 2009.

Aftel, Mandy. *The Story of Your Life: Becoming the Author of Your Experience.* NY: Simon & Schuster, 1997.

Baldwin, Christina. *Storycatcher: Making Sense of Our Lives Through the Power and Practice of Story.* Novato, CA: New World Library, 2007.

Cameron, Julia. *The Right to Write.* NY: Tarcher/Putnam, 1998.

De Salvo, Louise. *Writing as a Way of Healing.* N.Y: HarperCollins, 1999.

Dillard, Annie. *The Writing Life.* NY: Harper and Row, 1989.

Fox, John. *Poetic Medicine; The Healing Art of Poem-Making.* NY: Tarcher/Putnam, 1997.

Fox, John. *Finding What You Didn't Lose: Expressing Your Truth and Creativity through Poem-Making.* NY: A Tarcher/Putnam Book, 1995.

Freedom Writers with Erin Gruwell. *The Freedom Writers Diary: How A Teacher & 150 Teens Used Writing to Change Themselves and the World Around Them*. NY: Broadway Books, 2006.

Gendler, J. Ruth. *The Book of Qualities*. NY: Harper Paperbacks, 1988.

Goldberg, Natalie. *Writing Down the Bones*. Boston, MA: Shambhala, 1986.

Jacobs, Beth. *Writing for Emotional Balance: A Guided Journal to Help You Manage Overwhelming Emotions*. Oakland, CA: New Harbinger Press, 2005.

Jamison, Kay Redfield. *An Unquiet Mind: A Memoir of Moods and Madness*. NY: Knopf, 1995.

Joselow, Beth Baruch. *Working Without the Muse: 50 Beginning Exercises for the Creative Writer*. Brownsville, OR: Story Line Press, 1995.

Kominars, Shepard B. *Write for Life: Healing Body, Mind and Spirit through Journal Writing*. Cleveland, OH: Cleveland Clinic Press, 2007.

Lamott, Anne. *Bird by Bird: Some Instructions on Writing and Life*. NY: Pantheon, 1994.

Lombardo, Tom. *After Shocks: The Poetry of Recovery for Life-Shattering Events*. Atlanta, GA: Sante Lucia Books, 2008.

Manning, Marsha. *Undercurrents: A Life Beneath the Surface*. San Francisco, CA: HarperSan Francisco, 1994.

Marra, Reggie. *Living Poems, Writing Lives: Spirit, Self and the Art of Poetry*. NY: Xlibris, 2002.

Metzger, Deena. *Writing for Your Life*. NY: HarperOne, 1992.

Myers, Jack E. The Portable Poetry Workshop. Belmont, CA: Wadsworth Publishing, 2004.

Myers, Linda Joy. *Becoming Whole: Writing Your Healing Story*. San Diego, CA: Silver Threads, 2003.

Pennebaker, James W. *Opening Up; The Healing Power of Expressing Emotions*. London: Guilford Press, 1997.

Pennebaker, James W. *Writing to Heal: A Guided Journal for Recovering from Trauma and Emotional Upheaval*. Oakland, CA: New Harbinger Publications, 2004.

Rainer, Tristine. *Your Life as Story*. NY: Tarcher/Putnam, 1998.

Rico, Gabriele Lusser. *Pain and Possibility; Writing Your Way through Personal Crisis.* NY: Jeremy P. Tarcher, Inc., 1991.

Schaefer, Elizabeth Maynard. *Writing through the Darkness: Easing Your Depression with Paper and Pen.* Berkeley, CA: Celestial Arts, 2007.

Schneider, Pat. *Writing Alone and With Others.* NY: Oxford University Press, 2003.

Styron, William. *Darkness Visible: A Memoir of Madness.* NY: Random House, 1990.

Ueland, Brenda. *If You Want to Write: A Book about Art, Independence and Spirit.* Saint Paul: MN: Graywolf Press, 1997.

Weldon, Michele. *Writing to Save Your Life; How to Honor Your Story through Journaling.* Center City, MN: Hazelden, 2003.

Recommended Readings for Helping Professionals:

Anderson, Charles M., and Marion M. MacCurdy, Eds. *Writing and Healing: Toward an Informed Practice.* Urbana, Illinois, National Council of Teachers of English, 1999.

Chavis, Geri Giebel & Lila Weisberger, Eds. *The Healing Fountain: Poetry Therapy for Life's Journey.* St. Cloud, MN: North Star Press of St. Cloud, 2003.

Hynes, Arleen McCarty & Mary Hynes Berry. *Biblio/Poetry Therapy: The Interactive Process.* St. Cloud, MN: North Star Press of St. Cloud, Inc., 1994.

Leedy, Jack J., Ed. *Poetry As Healer: Mending the Troubled Mind.* NY: Vanguard Press, 1985 (out of print; available only from The National Association for Poetry Therapy).

Lepore, Stephen J. & Joshua M. Smyth. *The Writing Cure: How Expressive Writing Promotes Health and Emotional Well-Being.* Washington, D.C.: APA, 2002.

Lerner, Arthur, Ed. *Poetry in the Therapeutic Experience.* St. Louis, MO: MMB Music, 1994.

Mazza, Nicholas. *Poetry Therapy: Theory and Practice*. Oxford, U.K.: Routledge, 2003.

Mehl-Madrona, Lewis. *Narrative Medicine: The Use of History and Story in the Healing Process*. Rochester, VT: Bear & Company, 2007.

Mirriam-Goldberg, Caryn & Janet Tallman, Eds. *The Power of Words*. Keane, NH: Transformative Language Arts Press, in cooperation with Mammoth Publications, 2007.

Thompson, Kate, and Kathleen Adams, Eds. *Expressive Writing Counseling and Healthcare*. New York, NY: Rowman and Littlefield Publishers, 2015. This is one volume of a groundbreaking series called: "It's Easy to W.R.I.T.E."

Resources:

The Creative Righting Center. Director, Dr. Sherry Reiter. 718-998-4572. www.thecreativerightingcenter.com Poetry therapy training in New York and for distance learners. Lectures, seminars and individual therapy. The mission is "achieve wellness and emotional balance through writing, poetry, story and voice."

The National Association for Poetry Therapy. 1-888-498-1843 or for quick assistance e-mail naptaadmin@poetrytherapy.org This membership organization features an annual conference and networking for all persons interested in using the language arts for healing and growth. Members also recieve Journal of Poetry Therapy as well as museletters.

The National Federation for Biblio/Poetry Therapy. www.nfbpt.com e-mail: admin@nfbpt.com This is the national standards-setting body for biblio/poetry therapy since 1982. At the time of this printing, poetry therapy licenses exist in five states.

Internet Resources

http://news.utexas.edu/2011/08/01/pennebaker_word_choice The words people use are as revealing as fingerprints according to the research of the University of Texas Professor Dr. James W. Pennebaker.

Maryellen.Bova@wcsdny.org "Find Your Write Self." Maryellen Bova is a writer and educator who encourages her students to embark on a journey of self-nurturance and personal growth.

writeoutofdepression.blogspot.com Elizabeth Maynard Schaefer's blog contains writing prompts and other resources.

www.allthingshealing.com An on-line community for healing mind, body, spirit, planet.

www.bridgerossings.org Director, Lila Weisberger. Facilitates on-line seminars and workshops in poetry therapy and related topics.

www.creativewritingprompts.com Features more than 300 writing prompts.

www.editred.com Get peer critiques, publishing tips, connections with publishers.

www.favoritepoem.org features American saying the poems they love best. Incredible project!

www.goddard.edu/people/caryn-mirriam-goldberg Caryn Mirriam-Goldberd is the director of Goddard College's Transformative Language Arts Program, the author of nineteen books,and poet laureate of Kansas from 2009 to 2013.

www.healingstory.org The Healing Story Alliance, a special interest group of the National Storytelling Network, shares experience to inform, inspire, nurture and heal via story.

www.iajw.org International Association for Journal Writers To deepen, expand and juice up your memoir writing. Members access, classes, articles, and teleseminars.

www.inkwings.com A look at Linda Lanza's concepts of applying expressive writing in daily life for strength, growth, and healing. Includes bio, chapbook, inspirational quotations, and essays about finding meaning through imagination.

www.journaltherapy.com Director, Kathleen Adams. The mission is "to make the healing art of journal writing accessible to all who desire self-directed change."

www.loc.gov/poetry/180 This site offers a poem a day for 180 school days of high school.

www.maryreynoldsthompson.com Live your wild soul story through the language of poetry, metaphor, and nature.

www.myspace.com/afrikanamadonna   Barbara Bethea as poetess "Afrikana Madonna" for *Like Manna for the Soul* CD and upcoming book. First African American Licensed Registered Poetry Therapist, women's ministries.

www.nabsinc.org National Association of Black Storytellers promotes and perpetuates the oral tradition that embodies history, heritage, and culture of African Americans.

www.oncolink.com (Click on Coping and Search for Poetry). Alysa Cummings, Oncolink Poet-In-Residence. Greetings from Cancerland columnist, survivor poetry and poetry therapy projects.

www.pw.org. Poets and Writers This site includes literary press databases, contests and job info.

www.peerspirit.com Life and Leadership through spirit, quest, and story, co-founded by Christina Baldwin and Ann Linnea, offering writing workshops and wilderness quests.

www.poetrypoetry.com An audio poetry site with information and excellent links.

www.poeticmedicine.org Director, John Fox, CPT. The Institute for Poetic Medicine. "It's vision is to awaken the creative and healing voice in the human spirit." Check out this excellent DVD available from PBS: *Healing Words: Poetry and Medicine*

www.poets.org The Academy of American Poets. Features Online Poetry Classes, Audio Life/Lines, essays, discussion forums, biannual literary journal and free e-letters.

www.sherryreiter.blogspot.com An array of articles, poetry and writings on healing.

www.storycatcher.net The Storycatcher Network is directed by Christina Baldwin.

www.storyhelp.com The Center for Autobiographic Studies, directed by Tristine Rainer, focuses on the creation, appreciation and preservation of autobiographical works.

www.twc.org or info@twc.org Teachers and Writers. Resources for teachers and writers in education.

www.writersdigest.com Online workshops, prompts, and "101 Best Websites for Writers."

www.writingawaythedemons Links to authors' websites and tips on writing.

To arrange a workshop or lecture with Dr. Reiter and/or authors, contact us at www.writingawaythedemons.com or sherryreiter@yahoo.com
We welcome your comments and questions.

Sherry Reiter, PhD, director of The Creative "Righting" Center, is a licensed clinical social worker (LCSW), a registered poetry therapist (PTR-M/S), and registered drama therapist (RDT-BCT). Dr. Reiter entwines talk therapy with writing therapy; poetry, story, and the reclaiming of voice are dynamic healing components in her work.

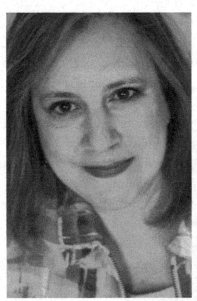

Photo by Elle Tyler

Sherry divides her time between writing, teaching at Touro College and Hofstra University, and private practice. At The Creative "Righting" Center, she mentors helping professionals who want to incorporate creative techniques into their work. Sherry is the coordinator of Poets-Behind-Bars, an innovative long-distance training program, in which poetry therapy trainees mentor inmates of the Indiana State Maximum Security Prison.

Dr. Reiter served as president of the National Association for Poetry Therapy (1993-1995), and was president of the National Federation for Biblio/Poetry Therapy (1995-2005). She is the recipient of the Art Lerner Pioneer Award (2005), and the Morris Morrison Education Award (2007) for excellence in teaching and bringing poetry to marginalized populations. Sherry aspires to the beautiful words of poet Dawna Markova:

> to live so that which comes to us as seed
> goes to the next as blossom
> and that which comes to us as blossom
> goes on as fruit.